SEX, LIES AND AIDS

Critical Praise for 'Words Like Freedom'

'...fully lives up to its promise of melding the voices of a single untouchable agricultural family in a UP village with a broad analysis of India's political economy.'

Krishna Raj, Editor
The Economic & Political Weekly

'Deeply illuminating. (India's poverty is) seen in concrete detail and vividly real by remarkable descriptive skill.'

Amartya Sen, Nobel Laureate

'A most extraordinary achievement...Academically grounded, yet immensely readable, it brings to life the experience of those whose tale has hitherto been swallowed up in the dark allusive term "masses"...makes all the recently published, highly praised novels on India look contrived and artificial.'

Jeremy Seabrook, Author of *In the Cities of the South*

'An extraordinary study of the human dimensions of poverty and development. Destined to become a classic.'

Shashi Tharoor, author of
The Great Indian Novel and
India: Midnight to Millennium

'A sensitive, ideology-free analysis of the poor and their history that stands out for its boldness and narrative accuracy.'

Outlook

'A fine biography... (will leave) an indelible mark on (a reader's) conscience.'

India Today

'Compelling... The voices of the poor are urgent, sombre, stoic and pensive.'

The Times of India

'A skilful melding of oral testimony and explanatory text.'

The Indian Express

'Not just the story of one family but the story of the masses of the Indian people.'

The Financial Express

SEX, LIES AND AIDS

Siddharth Dube

Illustrations by
Mario Miranda

HarperCollins *Publishers* India

HarperCollins *Publishers* India Pvt Ltd
7/16 Ansari Road, Daryaganj, New Delhi 110 002

Published 2000 by
HarperCollins *Publishers* India

ISBN 81-7223-409-0

Typeset in 11 pts Classical Garamond by
Nikita Overseas Pvt Ltd
19-A, Ansari Road, Daryaganj
New Delhi 110 002

Printed in India by
Gopsons Papers Ltd
A-14, Sector 60
Noida 201 301

To
Pratap and Savitri,
for their very great courage;

to
Brinda, Nilita and Pichaya
for being my home;

and most, to
Siddhartha Gautam,
for his brave and brilliant life.

Contents

Acknowledgements

My greatest debt is to the many Indians with HIV/AIDS who, over the past decade, have shared their stories with me, despite their own sickness, exhaustion and fears. For reasons of privacy, I cannot name them individually, but this does not diminish my admiration for them nor my gratitude.

I also want to thank my father Basant and brother Bharat because this book, like the one before, couldn't have been written without them. And for their advice, support and wonderful friendship, I thank Sohaila Abdulali, Tonuca Basu, Alejandro Bonet, Gitu and Pia Chugani, Rosemary George, Kusum Gupta, Gray Handley, Shilpa Hingorani, Vidur Kapur, Saleem Kidwai, Vageesh Naik, Neville Nagarwalla, Rosemary Romano and Kamala Visweswaran. And, not least, I have to thank my godchildren Anjali, Inaya, Itiya and Riyaaz for the great joy they give me.

No less, I want to warmly thank Denis Broun and Amartya Sen for their unstinting encouragement; Geetanjali Misra (and the Ford Foundation itself) for invaluable support; Michael Reich and the Harvard School of Public Health for the fellowship that enabled me to study there many years ago; and, not least, Renuka Chatterjee and Sheela Reddy for being superlative editors.

I would like to gratefully acknowledge the following people for having generously shared of their knowledge and experience. Their help was critical to researching and writing this book. Obviously, they do not necessarily share my views.

For their extraordinary help I am deeply grateful to Anjali Gopalan and her colleagues at the Naz Foundation India in Delhi; Drs Suniti Solomon and N. Kumarasamy of YRG Care in Chennai; Dr Subhash Hira and his colleagues at the AIDS Research and Control Centre in Mumbai; and Swarup Sarkar at UNAIDS in Delhi.

At UNAIDS, I would also like to thank Jim Sherry, Gordon Alexander and Pradeep.

At the World Bank, Prabhat Jha and, especially, Salim Habayeb. Vidhya R. Ganesh, then with DFID, for her incisive analysis.

In Chennai, Shyamla Nataraj of the Society for AIDS Awareness and Prevention; Dr P. Krishnamurthy of USAID's AIDS Prevention and Control Project; S. Ramasundaram (IAS) and K. Allaudin (IAS) of the Tamil Nadu State AIDS Control Society; Rama Pandiyan, D. Noorie, Shivananda and Ashok Pillai of INP+; and especially, S.Sekhar of Ambu Illam.

In Mumbai, Mandip Dhalawar and Sandeep Dadwal of the Lawyers Collective HIV/AIDS Unit; Medha Gadgil (IAS) of the Maharashtra State AIDS Control Society; and Radhika Ramasubban of the Centre for Science and Technological Change.

In Calcutta, Dr Asha Rao of the Bhoruka Public Welfare Trust; Dr Smarajit Jana of the All India Institute of Hygiene and Public Health; Trilochan Singh (IAS) of the West Bengal State AIDS Cell; and Dr Sekhar Chakrabarti of the National Institute of Cholera and Enteric Diseases.

In Delhi, Dr Bitra George of Safdarjung Hospital's Model HIV Counselling Centre.

I also greatly benefited from earlier conversations with Dr Mira Shiva of the Voluntary Health Association of India; Chattrappati Singh, then with the Indian Law Institute; Dr Radium Bhattacharya of the Gujarat AIDS Awareness and Prevention Unit; and S. Sundararaman of the AIDS Research Foundation of India.

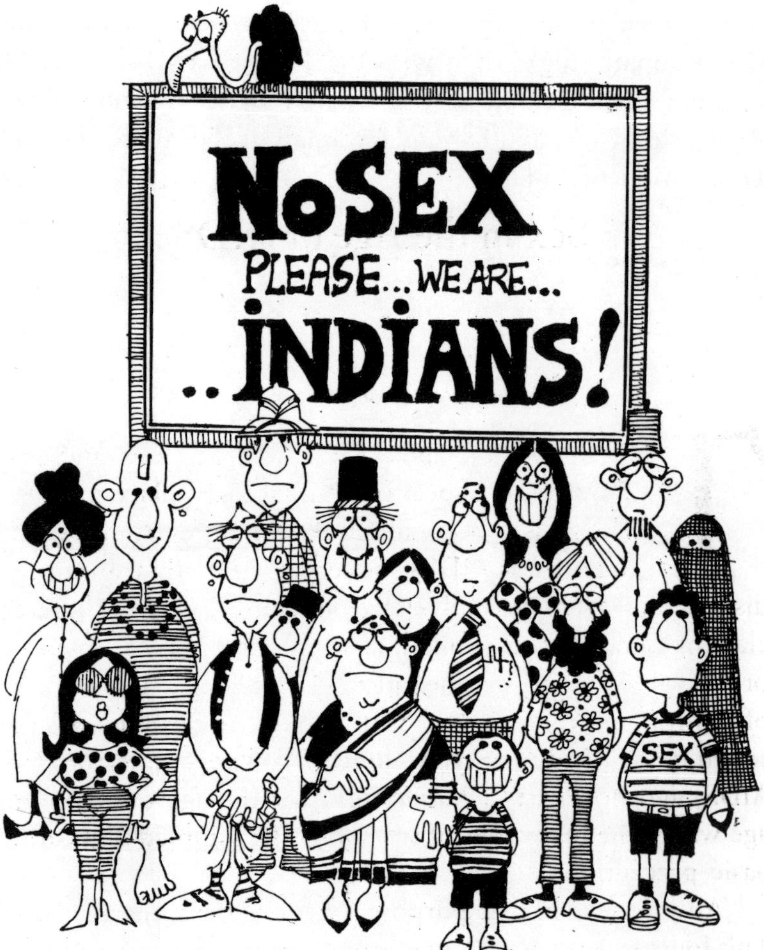
NoSEX
PLEASE... WE ARE...
..INDIANS!
SEX

Sex in the Age of AIDS

This is a book about sex, about Indians and sex, about every aspect of sex that takes place in India. And it is a book about AIDS. These things come together as AIDS is basically a sexually-transmitted disease and every sexually-active Indian — poor or middle class or rich, woman or man, aged fifteen or sixty, in school or college, working or unemployed — is increasingly at risk of contracting this disease. So this book is a romp through sex in today's India, a serious journey towards understanding AIDS, and not least, a *Kama Sutra* for the age of AIDS, an age where the many joys of sex should be sampled with some basic precautions.

All journeys have a purpose, or more than one purpose. This journey has three. A major purpose is to understand how we can protect ourselves — or our families or friends or adolescent children — from contracting AIDS as it becomes increasingly widespread in India. As AIDS is essentially a sexually-transmitted disease, most people who contract it are in their sexually active years, typically between the ages of fifteen and fifty. So, put bluntly, how can one have and enjoy sex without getting HIV, the AIDS-causing virus? As knowledge is power, this book is all about gaining the knowledge about sex and HIV/AIDS that we need to protect ourselves and other Indians from this fatal disease. One person dying of AIDS — a middle-aged professional — whose story is told in this book makes a telling comment: "I had heard about AIDS while I was in Mumbai. That it is a virus that kills you slowly. That you get it from sex. But one needs to have proper, detailed knowledge about what to do, how to protect yourself, how to have sex safely. It's not enough to know just a little bit."

The book's second purpose is to understand why India is today suffering from a severe and worsening epidemic of HIV/AIDS. This is what the best estimates show. About one per cent of all Indian adults are infected with HIV, about fifty lakh people. Every day another 3500 adults contract HIV. So are 1.5 lakh young children. In over half-a-dozen cities and towns, including Mumbai and Pune, three to five per cent of adults are infected, a dangerously high level. And AIDS has already killed another twenty to twenty-five lakh Indians. About 3.5 lakhs died last year alone. And because prevention efforts are very inadequate, there is every likelihood that within five years the number of infected Indians may soar to nearly four crores, or five per cent of the adult population at that point, which would be nothing less than a full-blown epidemic, on par with some African countries today. If so, by 2010 several crore Indians will have died from AIDS. So the book's third and very urgent purpose is to see what the government and we can do to prevent India from slipping into a catastrophic epidemic of HIV/AIDS; it is still possible to prevent this from happening if we act right away.

The best journeys are taken with a trustworthy guide. I promise to be this for you. As a health policy specialist and journalist who has worked on HIV/AIDS prevention in India and abroad for over a decade, I am probably technically well qualified. And I am open-minded and reliable. As your guide, I insist on just one rule. Journeys of discovery require travellers to go forth with open eyes and mind, so you must rid yourself of your preconceptions and prejudices. One very common prejudice to beware of is that some people got HIV innocently — a child, a faithful wife, or someone infected by a blood transfusion — and that others deserved to get it because of their behaviour — having sex before or outside marriage, going to a prostitute, or being homosexual. This prejudice is wrong, for every reason. As mortals, as people who are ourselves at risk of contracting HIV/AIDS (or suffering other tragedies), we must remember that every single person infected got it innocently, unwillingly, through no fault of theirs. Nobody, absolutely nobody, deserves to get HIV/AIDS. Nobody deserves to die prematurely and with such suffering. On this journey and later, we must respond with humanity and compassion, without bigotry or prejudice, to the huge numbers of Indians who have or will contract HIV/AIDS.

The journey that we're going to share is a sexual journey. Worldwide, including India, sexual transmission of HIV is responsible for eighty to ninety per cent of people infected. The other routes of infection are from contaminated blood and from mothers to their infants. So HIV/AIDS is essentially a sexually-transmitted or venereal disease like syphilis or gonorrhea, what we often call VDs or STDs. It is different from the other STDs only in that it is incurable, fatal and does not quickly produce symptoms. As sex is by far the most important route of transmission, on our journey we must frankly explore every aspect of sex. Heterosexual and homosexual. Between married couples or lovers or with prostitutes or strangers. Whether it involves vaginal or anal intercourse, oral sex, masturbation or kissing. We must discuss these sexual things openly, without discomfort, with the frankness and ease with which they are treated in the original *Kama Sutra* of two thousand years ago. This is essential if we are to understand how to protect ourselves and others from the risk of HIV/AIDS or to encourage government policies that help the larger public to lower their risks too.

Our journey is also necessarily a technical, scientific and medical one. We have to understand how HIV is spread, how a person can have safer sex to minimise the risks of contracting this virus, and how the illnesses of AIDS can be treated. Here are the essential facts needed to start this journey. (There is a detailed technical section at the end of the book, which you can refer to whenever you wish to know more about scientific or technical issues, even straight after this introduction.) HIV/AIDS is just a disease like any other. One must remember this. It is a mistake to think it is unique or demonic because it has no cure and spreads sexually. In fact, many other diseases have no cure or cannot be controlled by treatment — numerous cancers, for instance — despite being known to scientists and doctors for far longer than HIV/AIDS. Anyway, most people die from diseases that have cheap and easy cures: tuberculosis, for instance, can be cured cheaply but kills about one-fourth of the twenty lakh Indians infected every year. And there are and have been other killer sexually-transmitted diseases. From the sixteenth century till just fifty years ago, syphilis was incurable and maimed and killed lakhs of people worldwide, but it is now cured with a short dose of penicillin. Today, hepatitis B, also primarily sexually spread, kills nearly ten lakh people a year.

The virus responsible for AIDS is known as HIV — the Human Immuno-deficiency Virus. It was given this name because it attacks the body's immune system, our defence against disease. HIV steadily erodes the body's immune system and increases its vulnerability to tuberculosis, pneumonia, diarrhoea, tumours and other illnesses, which eventually kill the person. AIDS or Acquired Immune Deficiency Syndrome is the end stage of HIV-caused diseases. As AIDS is not genetic but spread by a virus, it is called "Acquired." And it is a "Syndrome" because people with AIDS develop a broad range of diseases.

HIV/AIDS is not an instant killer. For about six to eight years after infection with HIV, most people remain without symptoms and generally healthy; they are asymptomatic or HIV-positive. Because of the lack of symptoms, an infected person can unknowingly spread the virus to others. (There are simply no physical signs to show that a person is HIV-positive; only HIV-specific tests can confirm this.) After this long illness-free period, they begin to develop AIDS, and then — in poor countries like India where the average person lacks decent health care — it takes another six months to four years for the person to die. (Again, because they suffer and die from a variety of often common diseases, it is impossible to tell whether a person has AIDS; only trained doctors can do this on the basis of clinical symptoms, usually supported by an HIV-specific test. This is why most deaths from AIDS are rarely recognised or recorded as being caused by this disease, but are instead ascribed to the diseases that killed them.) Overall, in poorer countries, average survival is around eight years from initial infection with HIV to death. It is very important to remember that both HIV-positive people and those with AIDS pose NO risk to anyone through normal, everyday contact anywhere, whether at home, in office or in public. They need only to take precautions during sexual intercourse, should seek appropriate treatment for the mother to reduce the risks of newborns being infected, and should not donate blood or share injection equipment (whether for medical uses or for drugs) and take obvious precautions if they suffer from TB. So HIV-positive people and even those sick with AIDS can lead, and should be supported in leading, as normal and happy a life as possible.

Our journey is also an exploration of the aspects of Indian society that make the majority of adult Indians, whether poor or middle class or rich, very vulnerable to contracting HIV. One very powerful factor is our great discomfort with discussing sex. This leaves most Indians ignorant about sex and sexually-transmitted diseases, and consequently vulnerable to contracting HIV. There are too many other vulnerabilities. Poverty, illiteracy and the lack of even basic health care. The flood of single men seeking work in cities. The terribly low status of Indian women. The huge sex trade in women and young girls. The sexual abuse of street children. The violence and exploitation that the police inflict on prostitutes, street children, homosexuals and drug abusers. The inhuman laws and unfair policies that encourage such abuse. On this journey you must force yourself to unflinchingly see and understand these things, however harrowing: by doing so you will realise that preventing HIV/AIDS from spreading ever further and deeper into India requires nothing less than correcting these myriad and crippling disabilities.

And finally, our journey is an investigation. An investigation into why India today has the largest number of people infected with HIV in the world, when just fifteen years ago only a few hundred Indians were infected. An investigation into why the epidemic will almost certainly get far, far worse, with crores of Indians infected and dying. And an investigation into why our government and leaders have not done more to prevent this tragic epidemic — which will not just kill crores of Indians but also worsen poverty and perhaps imperil India's future — through the type of committed, sensible efforts undertaken by the governments of some other poor countries.

Before beginning our journey, I must make a brief digression. I have felt compelled to write this book because I have been a close witness, in the past fifteen years, to how HIV/AIDS has caused a *Kali Yug*, an apocalypse, in Africa and the gay community in the US. This book is my contribution in trying to prevent this catastrophe from being repeated in India. I have written it simply so that as many people as possible will be able to read it — in English or the several Indian languages in which it will soon be available — whether they are students, teenagers, young adults, parents, politicians, bureaucrats, housewives, shopkeepers, truck-drivers, teachers, business-people or in the armed forces. I have made it short as AIDS is an inherently depressing topic. And because preventing HIV/AIDS begins with talking comfortably about sex, I have kept the book sexy, a task made easy by Mario's uniquely provocative cartoons.

The first part of the book covers the beginnings of the spread of HIV abroad and then in India; the second part, the 1990s, during which HIV took on epidemic proportions in India; the third, the Indian government's inadequate response; the fourth and last part, the terrible devastation that almost certainly lies ahead, as well as the tremendous changes that are needed if we are to prevent this tragic future. In the first two parts do read closely the wrenching stories of the many Indians who have contracted HIV/AIDS: their experience, told by themselves, will illuminate many things about this disease and about why we Indians are so vulnerable to it. And read equally closely the first part of the annexe, how to have safe, fun sex — even the entire *Kama Sutra* — in the age of AIDS.

On with our journey.

The First Flames: 1986-1991

Two decades ago, at the very beginning of the 1980s, thousands of homosexual or "gay" men in North America, Europe and Australia began to suffer and die of rare diseases that only affected people with damaged immune systems. Because of its association with gay men, for a while this syndrome was called Gay Related Immune Deficiency or GRID. But researchers and scientists soon realised that this mysterious epidemic was not confined to homosexual men. The syndrome was also evident in hundreds of people who injected drugs or who had received blood transfusions. And most important, a world away in central and eastern Africa, thousands of heterosexual men and women were suffering from the same syndrome — the breakdown of their immune systems — which led them to develop diseases like tuberculosis and diarrhoea that are widespread in Africa, or occasionally even the rare diseases cropping up in the US and other industrialised countries. In 1982, this syndrome was given the name AIDS, Acquired Immune Deficiency Syndrome.

A virus called HIV

Putting together the pieces of this baffling jigsaw, American and French researchers eventually discovered that a virus[1] was responsible for destroying the body's immune system. The virus, moreover, was essentially sexually transmitted by intercourse between men and women or between men. Like some other sexually-transmitted diseases (STDs), the virus was also transmitted through both blood and breast-milk. Eventually in 1986, the virus was named HIV, the Human Immuno-deficiency Virus.[2]

Researchers also realised that because it takes about six to ten years for infection with HIV to lead to sickness, for every person sick with AIDS, there were many times that number who were HIV-infected but not yet sick. And for the same reason — this long illness-free period — it was clear that HIV had actually begun to spread widely from the mid-1970s, both amongst heterosexuals in Africa and amongst gay men in the Americas, Western Europe, Australia and New Zealand. Thus, the first cases of AIDS marked the emergence of the HIV/AIDS epidemic but not its beginning; probably about one lakh people were infected by the time the first cases

---

1 A virus is a tiny infectious particle. Measles, polio, the common cold and many other diseases are caused by viruses. Vaccines have been developed to prevent infection with these common viruses. However, there are no cures for any viral disease (including AIDS), only for diseases caused by bacteria, fungi and protozoa.

2 There are actually two distinct types of HIV virus, HIV-1 and HIV-2. But as HIV-2 is responsible for less than one per cent of infections, and because they produce similar symptoms, are detected by the same test and are prevented in the same way, HIV is commonly used to refer to both. There are also several HIV-1 sub-types, also known as strains or clades. The one most prevalent in both Africa and India is HIV-1C subtype, which scientists think may be particularly easy to contract or transmit sexually.

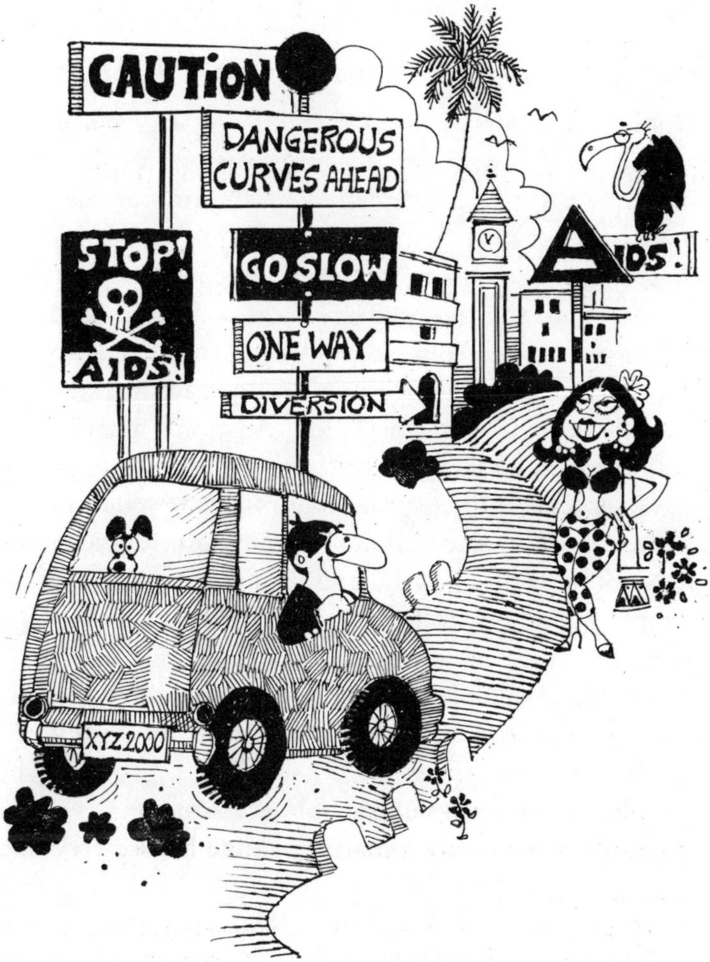
CAUTION
DANGEROUS CURVES AHEAD
STOP!
AIDS!
GO SLOW
ONE WAY
DIVERSION
AIDS!
XYZ 2000

were detected in 1980.[3] As reliable tests to detect infection with the virus were available by 1985, researchers were henceforth able to track how fast and where HIV was spreading. The availability of these tests also allowed individuals to learn whether they were infected.

Could governments have stopped AIDS?

Once researchers realised that HIV was primarily sexually spread, it followed that its transmission, as with all STDs, could be effectively prevented by the proper use of a latex male condom during anal or vaginal intercourse (or oral sex). So programmes were begun to encourage people to use condoms. In the rich industrialised countries, from the late-1980s on, gay men quite rapidly began to use condoms during anal intercourse and the numbers getting infected began to steadily fall. The Netherlands, Australia and a few other countries that established effective prevention programmes have succeeded in ensuring that only a few thousand people have ever contracted HIV. The US, Spain, France and others have done more poorly, ending up with lakhs of infected people and, until today, thousands of new infections every year. But in impoverished Africa, condoms were expensive and barely available, many people were illiterate and health services were weak, so HIV continued its deadly rampage.

In this modern world crisscrossed by tourists, business people, diplomats, sailors, soldiers, students, workers and migrants, it was only a matter of time before HIV spread to

---

3 Despite the many advances in the understanding of HIV/AIDS, scientists have not yet been able to satisfactorily pinpoint either the source of HIV or to explain why it exploded into an epidemic at this time. This is not as surprising as it seems: HIV is just one of over two dozen new diseases that have emerged in the past twenty years.

every continent and every country. Asia's first HIV case was in Thailand in 1984. India was not far behind. In 1986, the first case of HIV was reported in Chennai and the first case of AIDS in Mumbai, both being female sex workers. (As many prostitutes prefer to be called sex workers — emphasising that they are workers and deserve respect and workers' rights — this term is used in this book.)

If it was inevitable that HIV would appear across the globe, it was not inevitable that it had to infect thousands of people in the new places where it emerged. Certainly, it was not inevitable that these countries would develop epidemics of HIV/AIDS, affecting large numbers of their population. These tragedies could have been prevented if governments took sensible and resolute action. Scientists and health experts now knew what this disease was, how it spread, and how it could be prevented from spreading. Thus, most governments had a tremendous advantage over the nations of Africa or Western gay communities where HIV/AIDS had spread widely by the time the most basic details were known about it.

Tragically, India's government was amongst the many that failed to take advantage of this extraordinary opportunity. In the first stage of India's epidemic, between 1986 and 1991, about five lakh Indians contracted HIV because of the collective failures of our politicians, bureaucrats and health authorities. (By the end of 1991, more than a crore were infected worldwide, a 120-fold increase from 1980.) Later, through the 1990s, the government failed to prevent this first wave of spread from mushrooming into a widespread epidemic with lakhs upon lakhs of Indians infected. That story is told in the next chapter.

Havoc: Three hundred Indians a day get HIV

I was a journalist in Delhi in the second half of the 1980s, writing primarily about politics, but like now my overwhelming concerns were health and poverty. Even in those early years I was certain that the government would fail to prevent the spread of HIV, and that it was only a matter of time before lakhs of Indians were infected and we faced yet another enormous hurdle to progress. Why did I feel this terrible foreboding? Journey with me through these first five years to see why our government failed to meet its responsibility and the terrible consequences of this failure.

From 1986, when the first Indian cases of HIV and AIDS were discovered, the number of people in India testing positive for HIV began to multiply, mainly in Mumbai, Chennai and other urban areas of western and southern India. Each year the flood of Indians contracting HIV grew ever larger, as did the data from the centres that had been set up in many parts of India to track trends in HIV.[4] Soon, numerous HIV cases and some AIDS cases had been detected in every major city, and even from the larger trade, transport and pilgrimage towns in Maharashtra and Tamil Nadu. And there was widespread shock when government estimates showed that by

4 These centres make up the "HIV-serosurveillance" system. Samples of blood are tested that have been drawn for other reasons, such as from blood donors, people seeking treatment for STDs or tuberculosis, or pregnant women at clinics. The samples are not linked to personal information about the people — in other words, they are "unlinked anonymous screening" — solely to such demographic data as their age and sex. Typically, a serosurveillance system covers both "higher-risk" groups as well as the larger public of lower-risk persons. Pregnant women are taken as a surrogate or proxy for the larger public.

mid-1991 some five lakh Indians had contracted HIV.[5] Other estimates suggested twice that number or ten lakh people. Even taking the government's low estimate, between 1986 and 1991 nearly three hundred Indians contracted HIV every day.

The vast majority of Indians infected in these first five years were people whose sexual behaviour put them at high risk of contracting sexually-transmitted diseases: female sex workers, their customers, and men who have sex with men.[6] And because HIV is spread efficiently through infected blood, large numbers of those who needed blood or blood products for medical reasons or who injected drugs also contracted HIV. (Health researchers often use the term "higher-risk groups" to describe those whose sexual or other behaviour put them at greater risk of contracting HIV or other STDs.) Moreover, as many of the men with higher-risk behaviour unknowingly transmitted HIV to their wives or girlfriends, a large number of otherwise "lower-risk" women were also infected. To see how thoroughly HIV devastated people with higher-risk behaviours in just these five years, consider these figures.

---

5 Because India and other poor countries have very inadequate HIV-testing and tracking systems, only a tiny percentage of those infected show up in the government's health statistics. (This is true not just for HIV; India's health data is inaccurate for almost all diseases.) This accounts for the huge discrepancy between the small number of reported cases of HIV and the far larger estimates of people infected. It is likely that the actual number of people with HIV is more than hundred times greater than reported cases. Similarly, reported cases of AIDS are only a small fraction of the actual number of cases. This is for the simple reason that most AIDS cases are not recognised by doctors.

6 The term "men who have sex with men" is better suited to countries like India, as it covers not just the few openly "gay" men, but also hijras, male sex workers, bi-sexual men and the many men who have sex with other men but consider their sexual orientation to be heterosexual. See next chapter.

🎗 In 1987, just one out of hundred (or one per cent) of Mumbai's female sex workers were infected with HIV. By 1989, ten out of hundred were infected. By 1991, thirty out of hundred. And, by 1994, fifty out of hundred or every second one. There are roughly one to 1.5 lakh female sex workers in Mumbai, so in this one city itself about thirty to forty-five thousand of these desperately impoverished and exploited women and girls contracted HIV between 1987 and 1991. Sex workers in Chennai were infected almost as rapidly. And as prostitution is widespread in all of India's urban centres, including smaller industrial and trading towns, substantial numbers of sex workers in other parts of India were also infected.

🎗 Tens of thousands of their customers — men of all backgrounds and income levels — were also infected in this half-decade. According to one rough estimate, with forty out of hundred of Mumbai's sex workers infected by 1992, every night about two hundred men were contracting HIV in that city: seventy-two thousand men every year. In many developing countries, as in India, in the emerging period of an HIV/AIDS epidemic the majority of infections, half or more, occur amongst customers of female sex workers. This was confirmed by the data. The number of HIV-positive cases amongst men seeking treatment for other STDs, such as syphilis or gonorrhoea, at government STD clinics, skyrocketed. In Mumbai, less than one in hundred STD patients were infected with HIV in 1988. By end-1991, fifteen out of hundred had HIV; a year later, twenty-five. The infection levels rose quite rapidly elsewhere too: in Chennai, nearly nine out of hundred male STD patients by 1991, and in Vellore four out of hundred.

🎗 Also infected were thousands of men who have sex with men. Despite their great numbers, men who have sex with men are almost invisible in India. This is so because only a tiny minority of them, including hijras, are openly homosexual or "gay." Not only is there terrifying social prejudice against homosexuals but homosexuality, even between consenting adults, is a crime under Indian law. Under a colonial-period law — Section 377 of the Indian Penal Code[7] — homosexuals can be sentenced to life imprisonment or ten years' rigorous imprisonment. Because few Indians would be foolish enough to admit to a doctor or an official that they have sex with other men, the government's assertion that till end-1991 only eight cases of HIV were from homosexual intercourse lacked any validity at all. The true levels of HIV infection among men who have sex with men were not known. But a few small surveys by independent researchers reported that a large percentage were infected.

🎗 Large numbers of injecting drug users were also infected in these years. Injecting drugs, mainly heroin, is a significant problem in several northeastern states — particularly Manipur, Nagaland and Mizoram — that border the major drug-trafficking countries of Myanmar, Thailand and Laos. Drug use is also prevalent in universities and colleges, tourist resorts, industrial townships and the slum areas of major cities. Sharing of unsterilised needles or syringes is an extremely efficient way of transmitting HIV, with the virus carried by even minute traces of blood. So once HIV infects one addict in a needle-sharing group, others are likely to get infected at frightening speed. Of Manipur's estimated fifteen to twenty-five thousand injecting drug users, eight out of hundred were infected with HIV in 1989 but sixty out of hundred by 1993.

---

7 Actually, homosexuality as a sexual orientation is not an offence. An "act" of unnatural intercourse has to be proved.

- Also infected in their tens of thousands were women who were the wives or girlfriends of these men with risky sexual or drug use behaviours. Of course, almost none of the infected men knew they had HIV and so transmitted the virus unwittingly. Rough estimates suggest that about as many lower-risk women were infected in this period as people with risky behaviours. The increase in the number of "low-risk women" contracting HIV was seen in data from pregnant women whose blood was tested in antenatal clinics in urban areas. By 1990, thirteen out of every hundred women in Chennai had HIV, and nearly ten out of every hundred in Mumbai. As pregnant women are taken as a proxy for the larger public, this meant that 1.3 per cent of all adults in Chennai and nearly one per cent in Mumbai had contracted HIV.[8]

- And several thousand people who had blood transfused or used blood products such as immunoglobulin were also infected. Transfusion with HIV-contaminated blood or blood products has a ninety per cent risk of transmitting HIV. (Some others — both patients and, much more rarely, medical staff — were infected by poor medical practices in hospitals and clinics, such as re-using improperly sterilised needles or surgery equipment or being pricked by contaminated needles.) Because the demand for blood was far greater than supply and blood donation was not widespread in India, about half of India's blood supply came from poor professional "donors," who sold their blood to commercial blood banks. A 350 cc unit of blood earned them Rs 100 or so. But large numbers of

---

8 If anything, the use of HIV data on pregnant women as a proxy underestimates the levels of HIV in the larger public. This is because HIV leads to a reduction in fertility.

these professional "donors" were soon infected with HIV. Quite a few of these men worked as sex workers; others used sex workers, injected drugs, or were infected by contaminated blood-drawing equipment. By the end of 1989, in Mumbai ten out of every hundred professional blood donors were infected, with smaller numbers infected elsewhere. As the supply from India's thousand-odd blood banks was very poorly regulated and spottily tested for HIV, people needing blood or blood products were placed at considerable risk of contracting HIV.

Neglect and its toll

The lives of each of these five lakh or more Indians rapidly deteriorated into tragedy. I came to understand just how tragic when in mid-1991 I met scores of them while researching an article on HIV/AIDS for *Sunday*. This two-month journey across India was the most saddening one I had ever taken. In the worst-hit urban areas — Mumbai, Chennai, Pune, Imphal and other towns in southern and western India — HIV/AIDS had begun to visibly exact its terrible toll. The victims were amongst the most vulnerable and defenceless Indians.

In Mumbai, at an NGO-run STD and health clinic near Kamathipura, the city's famed red-light area, the woman doctor whispered to me in English that almost all of the dozen young women in the room were HIV-positive. They were all sex workers. Dressed in salwar-kameez or sarees and wearing only a fraction of the make-up they used back in the brothels, they looked no different from the housewives or teenage girls of this poor neighbourhood. None was older than twenty. The youngest, a fair, open-faced Nepalese, was just fourteen. Some were already sick with HIV-caused tuberculosis and other diseases.[9] But they could not stop working until they were visibly ill, said the doctor. They were in debt to their pimps and madams, knew that the police were in cahoots with them, lacked any employable skills, and had no refuge. On this wet June day, the small clinic seemed like any other crowded spot in the city. But to me it was stifling with the tragedy of these young girls.

The city's tuberculosis and skin diseases clinics were deluged with young men and women sick with HIV/AIDS. In one bed at JJ Hospital's AIDS ward, there was a young policeman, no more than twenty-five years old, emaciated, his skin bursting with boils. He was dying, sick with numerous HIV-caused diseases, including herpes, TB and chronic diarrhoea. Like many young Indian men, his first sexual experience had been with a sex worker and he had contracted HIV from this single, inexperienced fling. In the corridor outside, several young, sick and infected women, who were sex workers, were waiting for treatment.

Far in the northeast, in Imphal, the capital of Manipur, the city's main jail was full of hundreds of addicts — young men and some women — who had been arrested for injecting drugs (or dumped there by their parents), were then forcibly tested for HIV, and if found to be infected were kept in a group away from other prisoners. Consequently, everyone in the jail and outside knew they were HIV-positive. The jail authorities had no plans to ever release this group of several hundred young men and women infected with HIV. Not

9 In India and other poor countries with already high levels of TB, this is typically the first disease contracted by those with HIV/AIDS. Consequently, people with TB are now often suspected of having HIV/AIDS. This has worsened the fears and discrimination already evoked by TB.

because they had committed a crime that required lifelong imprisonment but simply because the state government had decided that they posed a risk to society. Neither the state nor the central governments cared a hoot that under India's laws their imprisonment was illegal. So day after day, month after month, these healthy young men and women sat in the jail's enclosed courtyard, usually motionless, heads bowed, like a herd of animals who know they are headed for the slaughterhouse.

In Chennai and Delhi, as in most parts of India, doctors and nurses were refusing to treat people with HIV/AIDS. This was true of both private and public services. Ironically, the premier hospitals with ample supplies of HIV-test kits were best placed to test people they suspected of HIV. If found positive, they summarily evicted them. Delhi's All-India Institute of Medical Sciences, set up to establish the best standards of medical practice, had turned away scores of infected people. So the beds in its small but well-equipped AIDS ward stood empty.

Outside these hospitals, there were people sick and dying of AIDS because they had been refused care. In a slum in northern Delhi, in a corrugated iron shack that reeked of illness, I interviewed a young truck driver who had been thrown out of a government hospital when a blood test revealed that he was HIV positive. "One morning all these doctors and officials came to my bedside, shouted at me that I had AIDS and that I should get out of the hospital at once. I kept crying but they just kept shouting at me, telling me to get out, that I would die for my sins. I first went to my parents' house in Punjab but they also threw me out. So for the last year I've lived here in Delhi. This hut belongs to an older friend of mine who is also a truck driver. He looks after me when he comes to Delhi. But my TB is much worse than last year. I am sure I will die soon."

Multiply the suffering of this handful of people by several lakhs: that is the total of the suffering caused by the spread of HIV in India in the first five years. Faced with such enormous tragedy, the only possible human response is to ask, when our government had the power to help save these lakhs of its citizens from contracting a fatal disease, why did it not do so?

From 1990 onwards, I searched obsessively to understand this life-and-death puzzle. That year, on coming to realise that I cared much more about health and poverty issues than about daily politics, I had quit being a full-time journalist and begun a master's degree in health policy at Harvard University's School of Public Health, in the US. In my search for answers, I took virtually every university course on HIV/AIDS. I read everything available on why the epidemic was flourishing in Africa, why it was finally being slowed in many rich countries, and why it was inexorably spreading in many Asian and Latin American countries. I interviewed and argued with scores of international and Indian doctors, health experts and government officials. Back in India, I sought out people who were infected, sick or dying with HIV/AIDS, or whose sexual behaviour put them at high risk of contracting HIV. On research trips to Kenya, Malawi and Congo in Africa — and to several Southeast Asian countries — I tried to understand why HIV was also soaring in most of these areas.

Three steps to an epidemic

Let me outline for you what India's government ideally needed to do, the strategy it needed to adopt. And contrast it with what our government actually did. In the huge chasm between these two approaches to HIV/AIDS prevention lies the answer to why lakhs of Indians contracted HIV in this five-year period.

By the late 1980s, learning from the relative success of Western gay communities and the failures in Africa, experts at the World Health Organisation and other institutions — and, no less, Indian health experts and activists — had a good understanding of how best to help people with risky behaviours not contract or spread HIV. By adopting the strategy and policies recommended by them, India's government, like other governments across the world, had a very good chance of preventing the initial spread of HIV and so squashing any likelihood of a future epidemic.

What was needed, as a first step, was to work constructively with those with higher-risk behaviours to raise awareness both of the behaviours that put them at risk and of appropriate prevention methods. To prevent transmission by the sexual route, awareness campaigns about STDs and HIV/AIDS, condom use and STD treatment[10] had to be energetically promoted for sex workers, pimps and brothel madams, and, no less, the sex workers' clients. These campaigns needed to be reinforced by face-to-face counselling, which is essential to changing something as deep-rooted and private as sexual behaviour. And the campaigns had to focus even more on clients, pimps and brothel madams than on sex workers themselves because sex workers are almost always powerless to push their clients into using condoms. Even today, many Indian sex workers don't even know what condoms are. And what are the chances of an abused woman, desperate to sell

---

10 Because the presence of common STDs, such as syphilis or gonorrhea, makes it much easier to both contract or spread HIV, their treatment hugely reduces the likelihood of HIV transmission. See annexe.

her body, being able to convince a typically drunk, lustful man that he should forgo the pleasures of "flesh to flesh" contact — which is why many people don't want to use condoms — and strap on a piece of rubber? Where they welcomed such support, sex workers needed to be offered alternative sources of employment or income.

Men who had sex with men needed especially sensitive awareness, condom promotion and counselling efforts that recognised that in India they typically had sex furtively and in fear. And given the great handicap of their addiction, injecting drug users needed a multi-dimensional approach, including access to addiction treatment centres, needle and syringe exchange programmes, education about sterilising or not sharing injections, and community support and employment opportunities.

Second, these and other vulnerable groups (such as the urban poor or migrant workers) required access to the facilities by which they could improve their sexual health. The number of government, private and NGO-run STD treatment centres had to be multiplied. At these STD centres and outside too, counselling and voluntary and anonymous[11] testing for HIV needed to be expanded. The counselling had to be of a quality such that even the most taboo sexual issues could be discussed and sexual behaviours made less risky. Ideally, STD treatment and sexual health counselling needed to be provided at even the basic levels of the public health system. (Of course, the public health system first had to be improved from its terrible

11 Given the great likelihood in India and many other developing countries that a person's positive result will not be kept confidential, anonymous testing services are the best option. Here, people are known only by a number and do not share any information by which they could be identified.

state.) Across all these services, equal priority had to be given to providing appropriate advice and treatment for women's sexual health needs; in India, STD services are overwhelmingly focused on men.

And finally but most important, it was already clear that all these elements had to be provided in a context where the rights of people with HIV/AIDS or with high-risk behaviours were respected and their needs put first. For instance, doctors and nurses had to treat and care for people with HIV/AIDS or from ostracised groups — for instance, sex workers or hijras — without discrimination. At the same time, public hysteria about the disease had to be calmed and the problem presented as what it was: just the spread of a sexually-transmitted disease that posed no risks of transmission by normal, everyday contact.

Obviously, given the unquestionable skills of India's bureaucrats, jurists and health experts, there was no logical reason for them not to recognise the great merits of this approach. In fact, the government had displayed its capacity for decisive action by establishing a committee on AIDS prevention within months of the first Indian HIV cases being reported. But I watched in dismay as from 1986 onwards India's officials rapidly adopted the worst possible approach to HIV prevention, far worse even than inaction. This was to treat HIV/AIDS as a law-and-order problem. The criminals were people with HIV/AIDS and those vilified as "high-risk groups." The government's reasoning went: these criminal people should be detected, forcibly tested for HIV, quarantined if found positive, and thus prevented from infecting blameless people.

The policies that emerged from this inherently unsound approach were a fatal mix of illogic, hysteria and force. In

1988, Dr A.S. Paintal, the then head of the Indian Council of Medical Research, the government's top advisory body on health, proposed that sex with foreigners be banned. Then, all foreigners (particularly Africans) and Indians returning from abroad were required to provide medical certificates attesting that they were HIV-free. Infected foreigners were to be deported; infected Indians jailed or quarantined. In the same vein, the National AIDS Control Programme recommended mandatory, forced testing of people suspected of "high-risk" behaviours. Sowing further prejudice and confusion, Dr Paintal announced that Indian women were "the reservoirs of AIDS." The hysteria mounted further in 1989 when Prime Minister Rajiv Gandhi's government proposed a law on AIDS prevention that would not only have provided legal sanction to such things as forced testing, but in fact would have given the government unprecedented powers. Thus, the AIDS Prevention Bill contained a clause allowing the government to "take such other precautionary steps to prevent the spread of HIV infection as it may deem necessary." In other words, any action taken by the government or its officials in the name of HIV prevention, however wrongheaded or unfairly damaging to a person, would have been beyond legal scrutiny; the government could not be held liable or guilty for it.

Fear, coercion and hysteria

Fuelled by these policies, HIV/AIDS-related abuse and victimisation multiplied across India. Police and health officials forcibly tested thousands of sex workers and drug users. Revealingly, the sex workers' clients were never touched. If they had, the police would have had to arrest innumerable politicians and other bigwigs, and no less, to turn themselves in. Those found to be HIV-positive or with AIDS were quarantined or jailed. In 1989, the government of Maharashtra deported several hundred Tamil sex workers from Mumbai to Chennai. In 1990, Tamil Nadu's government forcibly tested several hundred sex workers for HIV, and then locked up eight hundred of the infected women for several months. They were freed only because of legal action by civil rights activists and the mounting expense of keeping such a large number of people in isolation. Many other state and city governments also forcibly tested sex workers, though on a smaller scale than in Maharashtra and Tamil Nadu. In Manipur, hundreds of injecting drug abusers were forcibly tested and imprisoned. In 1989, Dominic de Souza, a World Wildlife Fund employee, who was gay and contracted HIV, was kept in solitary confinement for over a month by Goa's government. To permit this, the Goa government passed a law allowing mandatory testing of anyone suspected to be positive and the isolation of those found to be positive.[12] The Indian Railways banned people with HIV/AIDS from travelling on trains. Public fears and stereotypes were worsened by the government's AIDS awareness campaigns, which proclaimed that "AIDS equals death" or that AIDS was spread by "fallen women." The hysteria was stoked by sensationalised accounts by journalists that blamed sex workers and other "higher-risk groups" for the spread of HIV. They also irresponsibly publicised personal details of people with HIV/AIDS, including their names, photographs and addresses, leading to many

---

12 De Souza's mother, Lucy de Souza, challenged the act in court. She won a partial victory. The court said it would no longer be mandatory to detain positive people, except where the authorities felt it was a "justifiable" case. Mrs de Souza challenged this verdict in the Mumbai High Court, but lost.

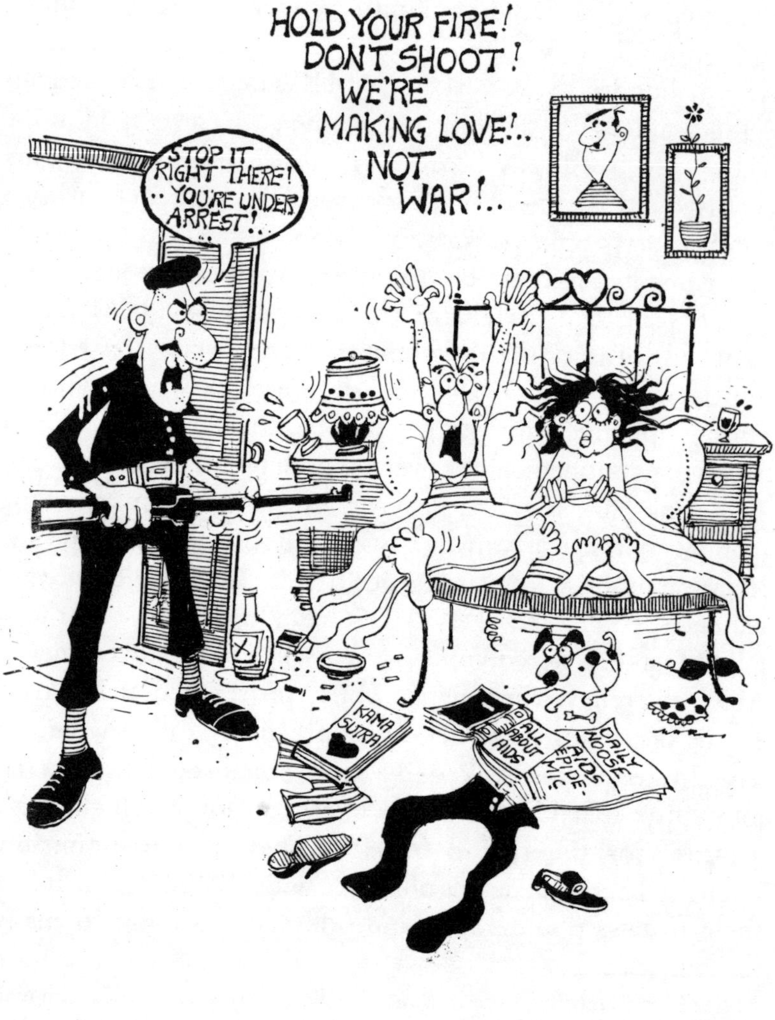
STOP IT RIGHT THERE! .. YOU'RE UNDER ARREST!..
HOLD YOUR FIRE! DON'T SHOOT! WE'RE MAKING LOVE!.. NOT WAR!..
KAMA SUTRA
ALL ABOUT AIDS
DAILY NOOSE
AIDS EPIDEMIC

cases of violent discrimination and even suicide. India's doctors and nurses were no less to blame. Despite being aware of the low risks of transmission to themselves, they refused to handle people with HIV/AIDS. This further stoked public fears about the disease. Even top doctors at the All-India Institute of Medical Sciences in Delhi denied treatment to HIV-positive haemophiliac children.

The policies of this period were also marked by a dangerous misuse of the concept of "higher-risk groups." This is a valid concept in health policy as it relates to HIV/AIDS and other STDs, reflecting that most people belonging to certain groups tend to have, by choice or circumstance, several or multiple sexual partners over their lifetimes. But the problem in India was, first, that the categorisation was not done with any scientific rigour, but was driven by the prejudices of Indian officials. For instance, men who have sex with men were left out, reflecting the untenable belief of Indian authorities that homosexuality is not widespread in India, that it is a Western import. The second error was even worse. Far from supporting these most vulnerable and "at-risk" groups, India's officials treated them as dangerous criminals. Finally, in practice India's officials focused their repression on the most defenceless of the "higher-risk groups," particularly sex workers, drug users, professional blood donors and some homosexual men. The men who used sex workers were spared, essentially because most of India's policy-makers were (and are) men and did not despise the many men who used sex workers anywhere as strongly as they despised other "higher-risk groups."[13]

13 The most blatant example of this bias towards the customers and indifference towards the sex workers themselves was the Maharashtra government's proposal, in 1994, to brand infected sex workers with indelible ink.

This approach of fear-inducing public statements, coercion, and victimisation of people with HIV/AIDS and of those vilified as "higher-risk" was bound to fail. Such policies had miscarried in every country that had attempted them.[14] In populous, chaotic and democratic India, these policies could never have been meaningfully enforced. Even if enforced, they would not have appreciably slowed the spread of HIV. Many Indians were married to foreigners, including the then prime minister Rajiv Gandhi. The scale of international travel by Indians — whether government officials, businesspeople, tourists, migrant workers or the armed forces — was enormous. Anyhow, HIV had begun to spread in India even before the first case was detected in 1986, and since then had essentially spread indigenously, from Indians to other Indians. Mandatory testing was impossible given the costs of the tests and the enormous number of people to be tested, let alone the insurmountable hazards of being able to correctly identify people with "higher-risk" behaviours or the legal and financial implications of quarantining huge numbers of HIV-infected people. And, as was to be expected, the government's policies only served to drive people with HIV/AIDS or with high-risk behaviours underground. Hiding from the police and health officials, they stayed away from hospitals and even from the government's STD centres. As a consequence, they were unable to learn about HIV/AIDS, find out whether they were infected,

14 There is some evidence to show that an approach based on mass forced testing and quarantine succeeded in quelling the spread of HIV in Cuba. But Cuba, an island with a tiny population, strong Soviet-style policing and few civil liberties — as well as universal literacy, excellent health care and a frank sex education campaign in schools — has nothing in common with India, or for that matter most other developing countries.

have their STDs treated, or change sexual or other risky behaviours in ways that would stem the spread of HIV.

During these years, apart from somewhat better screening of blood products, the government failed to implement any useful programmes, whether HIV/AIDS awareness, condom promotion or STD treatment. The five lakh or more Indians who contracted HIV between 1986 and 1991 paid the price for these failures.[15] No less, these failures also laid the foundations for the epidemic raging in our midst today. The development of sensible policy-making on HIV prevention was delayed by many years, just like Mrs Gandhi's forced sterilisation programme during the Emergency derailed India's family planning efforts for decades. The hysteria and discrimination also transformed HIV/AIDS from a disease, and that too a disease not spread by casual contact, into a cause of terror and discrimination. Several vulnerable groups, especially sex workers, who were the victims of grave abuses by the government were left deeply suspicious of the government. And the public and every sort of government official were left irretrievably hostile towards people with HIV/AIDS and of those they vilified as being "higher-risk groups." These two legacies of this disastrous period — suspicion on the part of vulnerable groups, and irrational

15 In this half-decade to end-1991, HIV multiplied widely within Africa, affecting an ever larger number of countries south of the Sahara. The number of people infected in most industrialised countries of North America and Western Europe increased steadily, though at a slower pace. Even greater increases occurred in Latin America and, towards the end of this period, in the Caribbean basin. And from the end of the 1980s, much the same time as in India, the number of people getting infected began to soar in Thailand, Cambodia, Myanmar, Malaysia and Laos, particularly amongst "higher-risk groups."

fears about HIV/AIDS on the part of officials and the public — have crippled prevention programmes.

Why did India's government adopt this disastrous, wrong-headed approach? As I understand it, India's officials — whether politicians, bureaucrats and health authorities — embraced this approach out of a complex and irrational mix of factors. Much the same reasons drove governments in many other countries, for instance Thailand, to adopt similar policies, with equally disastrous results. Fears about this new and fatal disease played some part. So did ignorance, as most of India's officials knew little about the sexual behaviours of the mass of Indian men and women. And so too did their mistaken belief that coercion and harsh policing could prevent the spread of a sexually-transmitted disease.

But the driving factor was their prejudiced belief that HIV/AIDS was a disease of deviants, the marginal and the poor, a view they often privately shared with me in interviews. Because officials believed that only "worthless" people were being infected and that HIV would never affect mainstream Indians, they saw no reason to spend money on the awareness, condom promotion, counselling and STD treatment programmes that people with risky behaviours needed. The prejudice was so overpowering that officials assumed that only poor or low-income men used sex workers, blinding themselves to the obvious evidence that in India teenaged boys and men from all kinds of social and income backgrounds use sex workers. Some officials — again reflecting views held by many elite Indians — even felt that these "worthless" people were being justly punished for their promiscuity by contracting HIV, and that their deaths would solve India's population and poverty pressures. In contrast, essentially because they believed that unsafe blood was the only possible route of HIV transmission to the middle and upper classes, to which they and their kin belong, government officials invested disproportionately huge amounts in screening blood supplies for HIV.[16]

Shaken by the carnage that I had seen that year and deeply pessimistic about the government ever adopting the kind of policies that were needed, I wrote in *Sunday* magazine in August 1991 that "hundreds of thousands of Indians will die from AIDS in the next few years. The tragedy of AIDS in the worst-affected countries of Africa is set to repeat itself in India." Sadly, it was soon apparent that this prediction was coming true.

16 The government moved to make blood supplies safer only when a number of middle class women were given Rhogam, an immunoglobulin supplement, that had been manufactured with HIV-infected blood.

Fire in the Tinderbox Forest: 1992 to Today

India tops world HIV figures

Imagine that you live in a village by a large forest. Imagine that you realise that for some new reason a devastating forest fire is likely, which will certainly destroy the village and kill many people. Imagine that only a few other villagers also see that this is likely to happen. And then imagine that the others just scorn your fears, saying that they have far more urgent things to worry about.

In the past decade, I have often felt like this imaginary villager, one of a handful of people fruitlessly warning that HIV/AIDS is going to kill lakhs of us and devastate our society. Unfortunately, our worst fears have come true. HIV has spread like wildfire in India in these years, reaching a new milestone literally every other year. By the end of 1994, HIV cases had been reported from all but two of India's thirty-two states and union territories.

By end-1995, India was estimated to have the largest number of HIV-positive people of any country. By end-1998, about thirty-five lakh Indians were infected, and over three lakhs died of AIDS that year alone. At the very beginning of 2000, the best estimate is that fifty lakh Indians are infected with HIV: about ten times the number in end-1991, and one-eighth of the global total of people with HIV/AIDS.[1] Of the sixteen thousand people contracting HIV every day across the world, 3500 are Indians.[2] Amongst the nineteen countries of South and Southeast Asia, only three have a larger proportion of their populations infected.[3]

All estimates are from UNAIDS, the UN programme on HIV/AIDS. The government's estimates are lower.

1 Some analysts argue, persuasively in my reckoning, that the government's estimates are unreasonably low and that the number of Indians infected is probably closer to eighty lakhs. But even if the government's conservative estimates are accepted, the essential fact is unchanged: that an enormous number of Indians are now infected with HIV. In any case, the government's response and plans should be based on "worst-case" estimates for today and the future, not the most optimistic ones!

2 Worldwide, by end-1999 over five crore people had been infected since the epidemic began. Of these, about 1.6 crore have died. The number of people getting infected multiplies each year. In 1999 alone, about fifty-five lakh people contracted HIV. The greatest number of new infections are in Africa; southern Africa is now as severely affected as central and east Africa, which were hit much earlier. South and Southeast Asia follow next, particularly India, Thailand, Myanmar, Laos, Cambodia and Vietnam. Warning signs are evident in Bangladesh and China. The situation is rapidly worsening in many other parts of the world, including Eastern Europe, Latin America and the Caribbean. But in most industrialised countries, the numbers of new infections continue to fall.

3 These are Cambodia, Myanmar and Thailand. In Thailand, about 2.5 per cent of adults are infected; in Cambodia, over three per cent, and in Myanmar, the best estimate would be four to five per cent. If Maharashtra and Andhra Pradesh are taken as countries — a fair assumption as their population is greater than most Asian countries — then their HIV/AIDS situation would be nearly as severe as the third worst-affected Asian country.

Two of India's states — Maharashtra and Andhra Pradesh — are in the thick of true epidemics, with over two out of every hundred adults infected with HIV. Several other states — Tamil Nadu, Karnataka, Nagaland and Manipur — follow right behind. In over half-a-dozen cities and towns in these six worst-hit states, about three to five out of every hundred adults are infected, levels that mark a full-scale epidemic. These worst-hit areas are Mumbai, Kolhapur, Pune, Satara and Thane in Maharashtra; Namakkal in Tamil Nadu; Hyderabad and Guntur in Andhra Pradesh; Churachandrapur in Manipur and Kohima in Nagaland. And levels are rising rapidly in other states like Gujarat, Delhi, West Bengal, Punjab and Kerala, where nearly one out of every hundred adults is infected. In other parts of India — such as Bihar and Uttar Pradesh — rates of infection are soaring in "higher-risk groups" and it is only a matter of another couple of years before the infections spill into and multiply in the larger public. And the number of Indians dying from AIDS has snowballed as ever larger numbers of infected people fall sick. The best estimate is that twenty to twenty-five lakh Indians have died of AIDS since the late 1980s. About 3.5 lakhs died in 1999 alone. Inevitably, about 1.5 lakh children have contracted HIV from their infected mothers and will waste away in a matter of years.

AIDS enters bedrooms of the rich

India's epidemic has changed not just in the soaring numbers of infections but also in that it is no longer concentrated amongst those with higher-risk behaviours but is instead multiplying within the larger lower-risk public. The evidence for this is so clear as to have dashed the misguided faith of Indian officials that HIV/AIDS would never spread beyond those whom they considered "worthless" — the poor or those with higher-risk sexual or drug-use behaviours — into mainstream Indian society. India's officials have no longer been able to treat HIV/AIDS as a distant threat confined to desperate sex workers, grimy STD clinics and emaciated drug addicts; it has entered the bedrooms of people just like them, middle and upper class Indians.

The epidemic's move into the larger public began with large numbers of "lower-risk" women getting infected by their husbands or lovers who had, or once had, high-risk sexual or drug-use behaviours. Thus, by 1991, the government's data showed that more than one out of every hundred pregnant women in Chennai and Mumbai was HIV-positive, and in Pune just slightly less. The level of infections amongst this group — which is taken as a proxy for the infection level amongst all adults — rose rapidly. The fastest increase was in Pune. By 1992, nearly four out of hundred pregnant women in Pune were infected, and by extension an equal proportion of all adults. And by 1994, about 2.5 out of hundred pregnant women were infected in Mumbai and several other urban areas in Maharashtra and Tamil Nadu. Then, as the number and proportion of Indians who were HIV-infected increased, even those who had few sexual partners and no higher-risk partners became increasingly at risk of getting infected. For instance, by 1994, with about 2.5 out of every hundred adults infected in Mumbai, it was more risky for an average person (man or woman) in Mumbai to have unprotected sex with another "lower-risk" person than it was for a man to have had unprotected sex with a Mumbai sex worker in 1988, when about two out of every hundred of them were infected. Today, in the half-dozen urban areas of India where three to five per cent of adults are infected, only a minority of new infections are amongst people with higher-risk sexual behaviours. In Mumbai, for instance, the best estimate is that about three-fourths of new infections occur as a result of intercourse between people with lower-risk sexual histories. Less than one-fourth of new infections can be traced back to sex with sex workers.[4]

Similarly, by the early 1990s, there was also ample evidence to show what the most realistic health experts had always argued and Indian officialdom always denied: that HIV/AIDS was not a problem solely of the poor and that it was affecting Indians of every income level. The data on pregnant women was itself powerful evidence, as it aggregates women from all income levels, especially the middle classes. Medical staff also reported the rise of HIV/AIDS in the middle and upper classes. In every major government hospital in places like Mumbai, Pune and Chennai, by the early 1990s hundreds of middle class men and women were seeking treatment. Blood samples sent by elite hospitals for HIV-testing were often testing positive. Doctors specialising in HIV/AIDS care reported that their patients included industrialists, film stars, top businessmen and other wealthy people. Moreover, several surveys of people with HIV/AIDS had been completed by the mid-1990s, which showed that many infected people were well-educated (often with college degrees), and were from middle and upper income backgrounds, including business-people, bureaucrats, managers, professionals, school and university teachers, and skilled industrial workers. And, the vast majority of people joining "positive peoples' groups," support groups for people with HIV/AIDS, are middle and upper income men and women.[5] All in all, from 1991 on, there has been growing evidence to refute the belief that HIV

4 Personal communication, National AIDS Research Institute, Pune.

5 The largest of these is INP+ — the Indian Network of Positive People — with about three hundred members across India.

would only affect the poor and that the better-off would escape. If anything, the evidence now shows that no class of Indians has been spared, from the poor to the very wealthy. While poor and lower-income Indians have probably been worst hit, the epidemic has made deep inroads into middle and upper middle income groups.

Why Indians are more vulnerable

How did we get to this state when the first cases of HIV/AIDS were detected in India only fourteen years ago? What is it about Indian society that makes most of us Indians, irrespective of class or background, so vulnerable to contracting this sexually-transmitted disease?

After having spent years travelling India's length and breadth, as well as working in or visiting about twenty-five other countries, I can only say that countries like ours are a tinderbox, a bone-dry forest, for the spread of a sexually transmitted disease like HIV. For innumerable reasons.

- Because we, like people everywhere, have sex.
- Because we do not discuss sex openly and so cannot even learn about life-threatening STDs.
- Because large numbers of Indians already suffer from other STDs.
- Because only a fraction of Indians have access to even basic health care.
- Because of the great scale of illiteracy and poverty.
- The flood of migration by single men between rural and urban areas.
- The terrible oppression of women.

These vulnerabilities compound each other so powerfully, and are so deep-rooted and widespread, that the vast majority

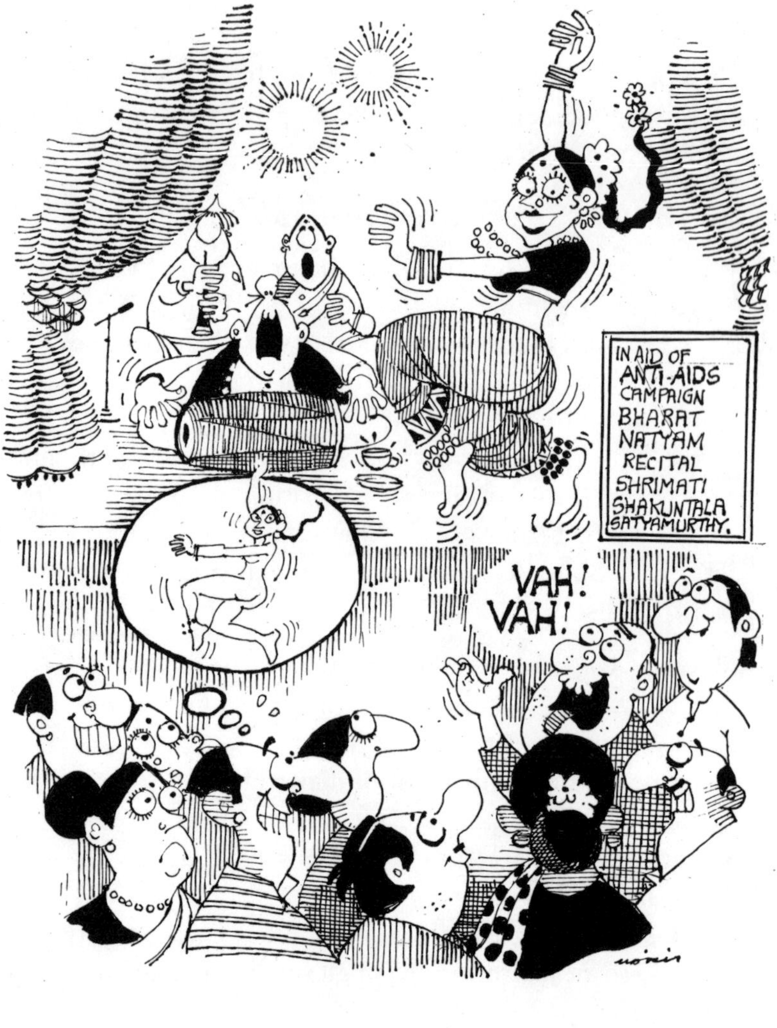
IN AID OF
ANTI-AIDS
CAMPAIGN
BHARAT
NATYAM
RECITAL
SHRIMATI
SHAKUNTALA
SATYAMURTHY.
VAH!
VAH!

of Indians are left too disadvantaged to be able to adopt safer sexual behaviours. Middle class, upper income and wealthy Indians suffer severely from some of these disadvantages, as is borne out by the many people from these classes who have contracted HIV. But lower income and poor people, both in urban and rural areas, bear the greatest number of disadvantages.

The moral tag and its price

The official view is that we are a uniquely moral society, literally that Indians don't have sex. Virtually every Indian political leader, bureaucrat and opinion-maker whom I have interviewed or talked to about HIV/AIDS has asserted this as an unquestionable truth. They argue in all earnestness that Indian society is more moral than others, that the average Indian does not have sex before or outside marriage, and that this will protect India from ever suffering from an epidemic of HIV/AIDS. The denial would be funny were it not so dangerous. Thus, even in 1991 when their own estimates showed that about five lakh Indians were infected with HIV, India's top health decision-makers continued to insist that we had higher moral values than Africans or Westerners, and consequently that an HIV epidemic could never develop here. The then Union health secretary R.L. Misra told me that "considering our social and cultural values and traditions, I feel quite confident that AIDS will not spread as far and fast as in Africa." At the Indian Council of Medical Research, Director-general Dr A.S. Paintal added, "Nowhere else in the world is chastity considered an important aspect of a woman's life apart from India." Dr A.N. Malviya of the All-India Institute of Medical Sciences in Delhi, asserted that Africans were promiscuous but Indians were "of a higher moral order."

Their belief continues unshaken. Hence, in 1996 an MP from Bihar asserted in Parliament that "AIDS could never dare show its face in the land of the Buddha." (If you find their denial astonishing, consider that these same politicians and bureaucrats and elite also deny that most Indians are poor.)

But these leaders and the many others who think like them are absolutely wrong. Travel across India with your eyes and mind wide open to its realities and you will see that there is sex happening everywhere, across its length and breadth, from the Kutch to Kohima, from Kashmir to Kanyakumari. Husbands and wives, unmarried lovers, teenaged boyfriends and girlfriends: they are all copulating. Sex workers — whether female or male or hijra, child, adolescent or adult — are desperately hawking their sexual wares. There is homosexuality aplenty: men are having sex with men, women with women. Girls and women, and often boys and sometimes men, are being raped. Infants and children are being sexually abused. Indians are having sex in rural fields and huts, on the pavements in towns and cities, in tenements and slums, in low-income housing complexes, in plush bedrooms, in corporate boardrooms, in offices, in mantralayas and ministries, in the bungalows inhabited by the country's most powerful politicians. Hindi-speaking, Urdu-speaking, Gujarati, Tamil, Punjabi, Malayalam ... Indians of every tongue are having sex. Of every religion. Of every caste. The hundreds of millions of absolutely poor are having sex; as are the equally large numbers of the merely impoverished. So are semi-skilled and skilled workers. So are the low income and the middle class. And so are the thin ranks of the upper middle class and the rich. Accountants, agricultural labourers, airline stewards and stewardesses, army jawans and officers ... convicts, call-girls ... hospital staff, housewives ... peasants, policemen and policewomen, politicians, professors ... scientists, sex workers ... teachers, truck drivers ... undertrials, university students, urban poor, urologists ... one of the few things they all have in common is that they have sex.

Anyhow, even if it were true that most Indians were more "moral" than other nationalities, having just one or a few sexual partners over their lifetime, it would not automatically follow that India would be spared a severe HIV/AIDS epidemic. Just how severely a country will be hit by HIV/AIDS depends not just on the sexual behaviour of its people but on whether they are vulnerable to contracting sexually-transmitted diseases when they do indeed have sex. The distinction is straightforward. Are people empowered to have safe sex by learning about HIV/AIDS, using condoms, having their STDs treated, forgoing or being able to refuse high-risk sex? Or are they so disadvantaged, for whatever mix of reasons, that they continue to have unsafe sex that puts them at risk of contracting HIV? It is because the vast majority of people in rich "industrialised" countries, from Canada to Japan to Australia, are able to learn about HIV/AIDS and then to act on their knowledge that these countries have, so far at least, prevented widespread epidemics of HIV/AIDS. Until the early 1990s, HIV/AIDS was feared to be a "pandemic." Literally, a global epidemic that had the potential to affect every country equally. But this has been disproved. In most industrialised nations the number of new HIV infections have fallen because of effective prevention programmes. Clearly, it is not that the average person in these countries doesn't have several sexual partners in his or her lifetime. Consequently, by 1999, ninety-five per cent of the global total of people with HIV/AIDS were in developing countries. In terms of the disadvantages faced by the average person, India's realities are diametrically opposed

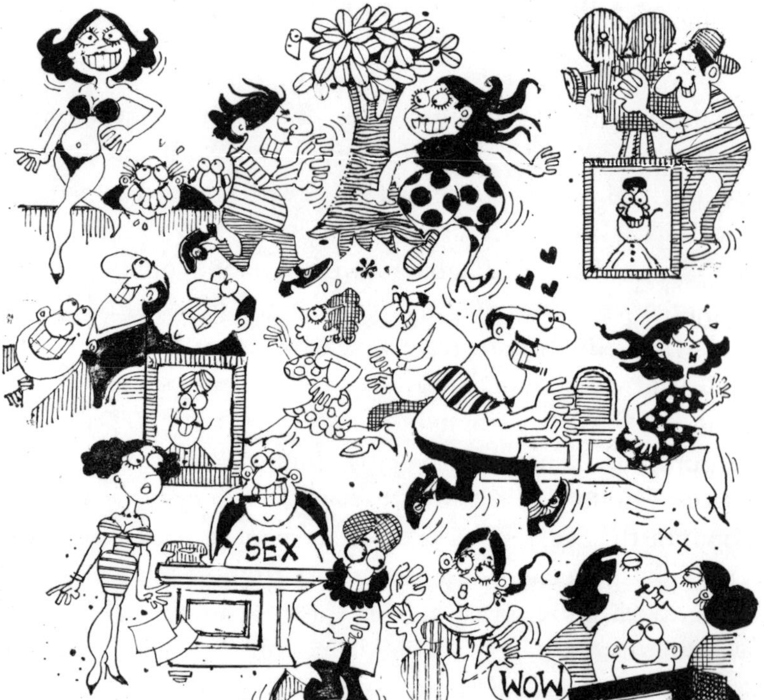
SEX
WOW

to those of these rich developed countries. Our realities are closer to Africa and other poor Asian countries. This is why in some parts of India, HIV has multiplied as fast as anywhere in Africa.

Prudes and prejudice

Our vulnerability to HIV/AIDS and other STDs is enhanced by our society-wide taboo on discussing sexual issues. The taboo means that there are almost no opportunities — whether at home, school, or through the media — for either the young or adults to learn about sexual issues or how to guard themselves from being infected by HIV or other STDs. Why else would such bizarre notions persist that a drop of sperm is equal to sixty drops of blood, or that masturbating depletes energy! Young people especially need correct information about sex as around half of all people who contract HIV do so before the age of twenty-five. But Indian parents, even those from our tiny Westernised minority, will not discuss sexual issues with their children. Or they will do so in ways that worsen fears and misconceptions. And conservative groups prevent sex education in schools or colleges, (even in such expensive, private schools as Mumbai's Cathedral) or even open discussion in the press. No less damaging, our censorship and pornography laws — adopted unthinkingly from our Victorian former masters — forbid, in the land of the Kama Sutra sexually frank advertising campaigns or explicit literature that people could learn from. The silence and hypocrisy is so powerful that even well-educated Indians, let alone the crores who are illiterate or poorly educated, know little about sexuality, often not even how to have sex on their wedding night or how to prevent STDs. And this environment makes it difficult for people to act on even what they know, for instance, buying condoms in shops or other public places.

This environment also breeds and perpetuates dangerous myths and superstitions. Indian men have begun to seek out younger female partners in the belief that they are unlikely to have STDs or HIV/AIDS. In parts of India, the myth still persists that sex with a virgin actually cures men of various STDs, including HIV/AIDS. And some of the government's HIV/AIDS awareness campaigns have been so shoddy as to generate fresh myths. One such dangerous myth, spawned by awareness messages that only depict or mention vaginal sex as a cause of STDs or HIV, is that HIV is contracted only through vaginal sex, and hence that it is safe to have anal sex, whether with a woman, man or hijra. Another is that STDs automatically lead to AIDS, a fear that has traumatised thousands of ill-informed Indians.

Poverty, the death knell

The consequences of the taboo on discussing sexual issues are most severe where the illiterate or poorly educated majority of India's people are concerned. For the half to three-fourths of India's adult population who are illiterate or poorly educated, it is very difficult to learn about HIV/AIDS. They cannot read newspaper articles or advertisements, leaflets or even simple billboards. They can learn from TV or radio, but even today only a small percentage of poorer Indians have regular access to these media. Moreover, because of oppressive censorship laws, sexual issues are almost never covered in depth by these media. The only avenue left for the poorly educated to learn about HIV/AIDS is to talk to each other, this being the major source of learning on many issues. But the taboo on discussing sexual issues prevents this. In any case, learning about HIV/AIDS from word-of-mouth is more often a way of spreading misconceptions, fears and prejudices than of gaining useful information. To begin with, almost none amongst the poor have access to reliable information on HIV/AIDS. And it is a very complex disease to understand, its intricacies baffling even well-educated people. If you were illiterate or poorly educated, could you understand — and then accurately explain to others — what HIV is, the routes by which it is spread, how other STDs increase the risk of transmission and infection, why infected people don't get sick for years? In fact, surveys show that even amongst Indians who have completed secondary school, misinformation abounds despite a decade of discussion and programmes about HIV. Only a small percentage know that condoms can prevent HIV transmission. While many of them are aware of a disease called AIDS and even that it is sexually transmitted, many think that it can spread from kissing, sharing utensils, or from mosquitoes.

Illiteracy is not the only aspect of poverty that makes people vulnerable to STDs like HIV/AIDS. Poverty in India is so extreme that very poor Indians — who make up more than a third of our population — cannot easily afford to buy condoms (even though cheap ones cost just Rs 2 a piece), find it difficult to use them because they live on the pavement or in crowded hovels or huts where privacy is impossible, and cannot afford to buy medicines, even for treating their STDs. Poverty is also the major reason why tens of millions of rural men leave their wives and families behind and migrate for months on end to towns, cities or industrial areas. There, these men, brimming with sexual desires, desperately lonely, exploited and overworked, ground down by the squalor, very often have sex with sex workers, neighbourhood women or other men. With access only to quacks for health care, they often suffer from multiple STDs. On going home they have sex with their wives, unwittingly transmitting HIV and other STDs. And poverty is the reason why street children sell their bodies for money, why the young "helper" boys working on long-distance trucks unwillingly agree to have sex with the drivers and loaders.

The government's lack of concern about the poor also means that the vast majority of Indian men and women rarely have access to the kind of health services where they could have their STDs treated, or learn how to prevent HIV or even about such a basic thing as taking good care of one's genitals. Which of us who has ever queued for hours at a government hospital or fruitlessly searched for a health centre in rural areas, does not know that India has a terrible health care system? In fact, India's public health services are primitive even by the standards of developing countries, both in terms of coverage and quality. In most Indian states barring Tamil Nadu and Kerala, many primary health care clinics exist only on paper, or have no doctors or nurses or medicines, or are open for only a few hours a day or even a few days in a month. District referral hospitals lack women doctors (to see women patients), specialists, basic medicines, diesel for generators, and are often so short of beds that patients who have just undergone surgery are made to sleep on the floor. Matters are scarcely better in urban areas. Municipal dispensaries and peripheral hospitals barely function, particularly as they lack medicines and other supplies. Anyhow they are so few and far between that most of the poor don't even know they exist. Even the large public hospitals do not offer the poor any relief. Doctors are so overburdened that they often see a hundred patients every hour. Everything is in short supply: staff, life-saving equipment, beds, antibiotics and vaccines, gloves, disposable needles, incinerators for infectious waste, even water and electricity. And corruption is rampant, with bribes often required for having a patient admitted. Of course, the miserable state of the public health services is not surprising as the central and state governments together spend just about Rs 70 per person annually on health; states like Uttar Pradesh and Bihar spend even less. Even this grossly inadequate sum is squandered by inefficiency and corruption. Worse, government spending on health has been drastically cut in the past decade of economic reforms.

Given the miserable condition of the public health system, most poor, low and middle income people turn to private practitioners. (The rich and powerful, including bureaucrats and politicians, are the only ones treated well at the government hospitals. Anyhow, they can also afford the best private health care, in India or abroad. Don't forget that our government spends many crore rupees each year to send a handful of senior Indian politicians and their families abroad for medical treatment.) Unfortunately, even after spending large sums from their own pockets, they can almost never find good care, only inappropriate treatment, unnecessary injections, and spurious or outdated antibiotics. This is because the majority of these practitioners — whether practising allopathy, homeopathy, ayurveda or unnani — are untrained and unlicensed. Certificates claiming that a person is a Registered Medical Practitioner (RMP) are easy to forge.

A death sentence for women

Another vulnerability greatly responsible for the ferocity of India's epidemic is the shamefully oppressed state of Indian women. The conditions of women in India are still amongst the worst of any society in the world, certainly far worse than in most African countries. Poorer Indian women are especially

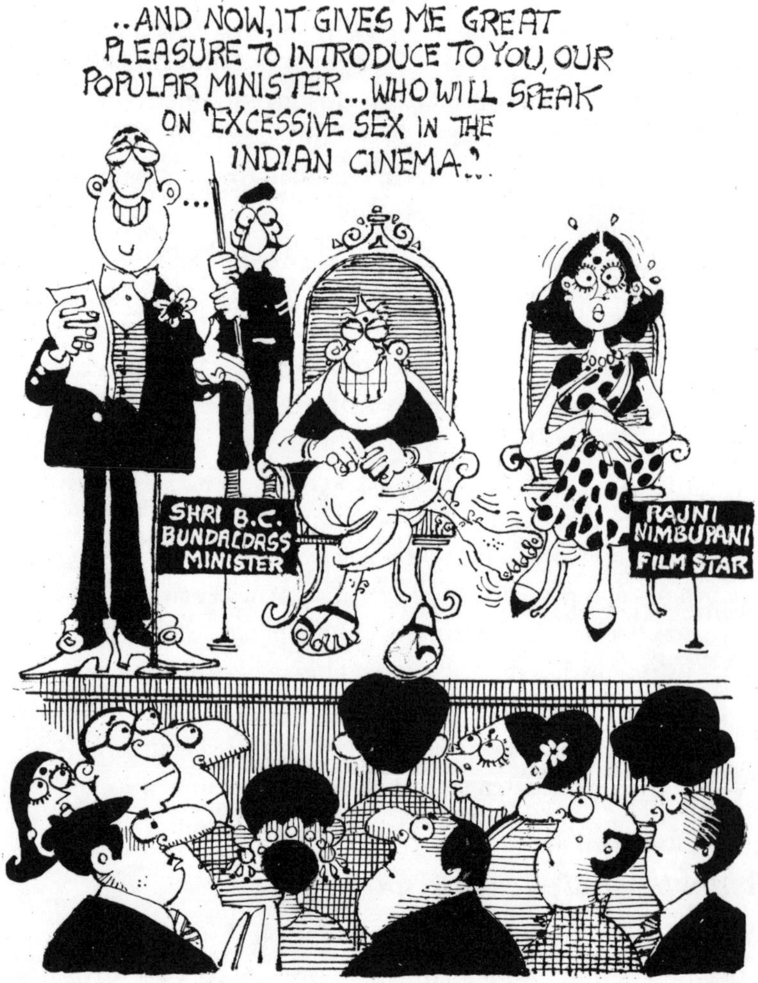
..AND NOW, IT GIVES ME GREAT PLEASURE TO INTRODUCE TO YOU, OUR POPULAR MINISTER ... WHO WILL SPEAK ON 'EXCESSIVE SEX IN THE INDIAN CINEMA.'..
SHRI B.C. BUNDALDASS MINISTER
RAJNI NIMBUPANI FILM STAR

vulnerable to contracting HIV. They also suffer from the multiple disadvantages faced by all Indian women. Consequently, huge numbers of poor or defenceless girls and women choose — or are forced by their families or by criminal networks — to become sex workers. Others turn to sex work only during particularly difficult periods of their life, or do it as a part-time job to earn money, otherwise working as a housewife or professional vegetable seller. Estimates suggest that across India about fifty lakh young girls and women are involved in sex work. Many lakhs more come from Nepal and Bangladesh. Many work in brothels; others ply urban streets, markets, bus stops and railway platforms; others, their homes in slums and chawls; others, highways or near their own villages; and yet others work as call girls from guest-houses and hotels in middle class and upper class neighbourhoods. Most of them are reduced to being modern day bonded labourers or indentured slaves, trapped in debt and terror by criminals who are in cahoots with corrupt policemen and politicians. But even the best paid are abused and exploited by the police and powerful men. Whatever their situation, they are rarely in a position to ensure safe sex. Hence, an Indian sex worker's occupation is, in the age of HIV/AIDS a death sentence. This is why more than three out of four of Mumbai's sex workers are now HIV-positive; amongst the poorest sex workers, who service more clients to survive, nine out of ten are infected.

The stresses on Indian women are endless. Many girls and women are sexually abused at home or raped outside. They are in no position to resist. Even if she is married, educated and not poor, the average Indian woman is dangerously disadvantaged in sexual matters. She is considered indecent if she seeks information about any sexual issue, even about how to prevent STDs. Seeking treatment for STDs brings shame on the family, even if her husband has infected her. She rarely has any say in whether she wants to have sex or not. She cannot require her husband to use a condom even if she fears that he has HIV/AIDS or other STDs. As a result, one of the largest groups infected with HIV/AIDS in India is that of monogamous women who were infected by their husbands.[6]

And because tradition dictates that men and women should not intermingle and forbids sex outside marriage, more than in most other societies Indian men have sex with female sex workers. In the age of HIV/AIDS, this pattern of huge numbers of men having sex with a small pool of sex workers has terrible consequences. The risks to the sex workers of contracting HIV are magnified, as they have sex with numerous men every day, any of whom may be HIV-positive. In turn, numerous men contract HIV from each infected sex worker. The upshot is that HIV spreads explosively. In India, men of all backgrounds and income levels go to female sex workers. Thus, it is a common practice — in some circles, almost a tradition — for the sons of middle class, upper class and wealthy families to have their early sexual experiences with female sex workers, often the more expensive "call girls." And armed with ample pocket money and the anonymity of big cities, many college-going and even school boys from better-off families now go to sex workers, either to brothels or to call girls. So too do men and adolescents from lower middle income, low income and poorer families, frequenting

6 Currently, in India, nearly twice as many men as women are infected. But worldwide experience shows that as the epidemic matures, equal numbers of men and women are infected, and then, as in Africa today, more women are likely to be infected.

the brothels that exist in almost every Indian town and city, or finding streetwalkers. Particularly likely to go to sex workers are migrant workers, as they typically only visit their wives once or twice a year. So too are those with occupations that require extensive travel or single postings, such as businessmen, politicians, bureaucrats, armed forces men, hotel staff, and those in transport occupations, whether trucking or in the airlines. And so do those men whose jobs bring them in frequent contact with sex workers, such as policemen. Hence, far from this being the habit of a few "deviants," it is clear that a large proportion of Indian men, of every background, go to sex workers frequently, and that even larger numbers go at least a few times in their lifetimes. The proof is the huge numbers and varied backgrounds of men infected with STDs and now with HIV.

Those invisible men who have sex with men

Similarly, both because men cannot mix with women and because so many of them are single migrants, very many Indian men have sex with other men, male sex workers and hijras. Just like the clients of female sex workers, men who have sex with men cover the whole spectrum of Indian society: ranging from the rich to the middle class to the poor, from politicians and businessmen to men in the armed forces and police to truck drivers to migrant workers. But despite their numbers and being drawn from every background, in India men who have sex with men are almost invisible. This is partly because the powerful prejudice against homosexuality and the family pressures to get married force many homosexual or bi-sexual men to get married, have children, and lead apparently heterosexual lives. And it is also because the vast majority of these men consider themselves to be heterosexual in orientation. Many assert that they have sex with other men solely as a convenient way to release their "heat" or sperm. Whatever their actual sexual orientation, all these men are at especially high risk of contracting or spreading HIV as they typically have unprotected anal intercourse. For physiological reasons, this is much more efficient at transmitting HIV, to both the receptive or penetrative partner, than vaginal intercourse. Condoms are rarely used because this sex is typically furtive and hurried, often taking place in public places like parks or toilets. And even when condoms are used, they often tear because these men do not know that extra lubricants are needed for anal sex, especially as Indian condoms are not very strong. (Saliva is not lubricating enough; oil-based products like vaseline, ghee or hair oil tear the condom.) And because many men insist that a man giving them oral sex ("blow job") not remove his mouth until after they ejaculate, the risks of infection from oral sex are greatly multiplied.

Overall, because India's population of men who have sex with men is so large and so much a part of "heterosexual" society — with many of these men having sex with women too, either with their wives or female sex workers — the rising levels of HIV infection amongst these men has fuelled the mainstream epidemic in just the same way as the spread of HIV amongst female sex workers. Unfortunately, the government's persisting denial means that there is no meaningful data on HIV/AIDS amongst gay or other men who have sex with men. The government's most recent estimate is that much less than one per cent of HIV infections are from homosexual sex. However, in southeast Asian countries where this issue is handled more frankly, between fifteen to thirty per cent of infections are attributed to transmission from men who have sex with men, and there is simply no reason to believe that the proportion in India would be significantly below this range.[7]

Given these multiple vulnerabilities, is it any surprise that at any time one in ten Indian adults suffer from STDs, which further multiplies their risks of contracting or transmitting HIV? Until the emergence of HIV/AIDS, STD control was simply not a priority for the government, with several crore poorer Indians left to suffer, unattended, from crippling and sometimes fatal STDs. The government's existing network of 372 STD clinics, many located in major hospitals, is so poorly funded that it lacks even essential diagnostic equipment, antibiotics and trained staff. Only a minority of people with STDs seek treatment at these facilities. But even those who do so get such poor treatment that their infections often persist. Those who seek private treatment are typically as badly off, as few Indian practitioners, barring expensive specialists, are trained in treating STDs. Consequently, most people with STDs simply buy antibiotics at chemists and treat themselves. They may find temporary relief but with little knowledge of their infection and of the correct drugs and dosage, their infection almost always persists and gets complicated. Indian women are particularly badly off, commonly suffering from untreated STDs that cause great physical distress and lead to infertility and severe long-term complications. For physiological reasons, women often do not have symptoms of STD infection and so do not seek

7 A recent study reports that one in ten "men who have sex with men" seeking voluntary testing in Mumbai are infected with HIV. Studies in Mumbai also point to an epidemic of HIV/AIDS amongst street children, largely as a result of sexual abuse and prostitution. In other parts of India, the likelihood that street children will be sexually abused or work as sex workers, and so contract STDs or HIV, is probably as great.

treatment. Even if they are suffering, they are very reluctant to seek care because of the great stigma attached to their being infected with an STD, especially if they have to seek treatment at centres known to specialise in STD treatment. Anyhow, even if they seek treatment for STDs or routine gynaecological check-ups, there are very few places for the average Indian woman to find adequate care. Even in urban areas, few public STD clinics have female doctors, male doctors do not examine women patients properly or provide correct treatment, family planning clinics don't treat STDs, and cheaper private medical practitioners are ill-prepared for treating these problems. For rural women, there is a virtual absence of appropriate care.

These myriad vulnerabilities, affecting rich and poor (especially the latter), explain why HIV has spread like wildfire in India. Of course, in a huge country with a billion people, there is some diversity in both sexual behaviours and the mix of factors that make people vulnerable. For instance, in the Northeast hill states women have a higher social status than elsewhere in India, men and women can mix and discuss sexual issues more freely, more people are literate, and fewer people go to work in big cities. On the negative side, however, is the widespread civil strife and the intrusive presence of the armed forces: these too often lead to women being abused or taking to sex work. Another negative factor is that the region is increasingly a smuggling route for heroin and other drugs. The easy availability of heroin has led many young people in the Northeast states to take to injecting drugs. To take other examples of the mix of positive and negative factors, while Punjab has less poverty it also has many of its men working as truck drivers, large numbers of whom have contracted HIV from having sex with sex workers on their transport routes. And in Kerala, while high literacy and better health services are a plus point, widespread migration by both men and women increases the likelihood of risky sexual behaviours.

Twelve portraits in the age of AIDS

In early 1999, I spent four months travelling across India as part of the research for this book, spending most of my time in the worst-affected western and southern areas. I was retracing my first journey of 1991, and two shorter research trips I had made in 1994 and 1997. That first journey had, until then, been the most saddening one of my life. But that sadness was nothing compared to the mix of despair and grief that choked me as I went from city to city this time. On the first journey I had met just handful of people sick or dying of HIV/AIDS. Now there were hundreds and even thousands from every income group ranging from the destitute to the poor, low, middle and upper income groups. To see this tragedy grip India was unbearable. Over the years, especially while researching and writing an earlier book on poverty, I had learnt to firmly keep some psychological distance between the tragedies I witnessed and myself. But the tragedies I recorded this time were so intense and jarring that after some interviews I could do nothing but go to my hotel room and cry. The visions of these tragedies — and the knowledge that even greater tragedies lie ahead — have been so haunting that I have not been able to prevent myself from sinking into prolonged depression while writing this book.

The dozen stories I relate of the many Indians with HIV/AIDS whom I met in these months will show you why. The stories of a young saleswoman, the owner of a flourishing business, a professional with a private sector company, a gay man, a housemaid, sex workers, an illiterate young labourer, and a widowed housewife testify that India is beginning to repeat Africa's nightmarish experience with HIV/AIDS. Their names and circumstances have been changed to protect their identities. They are testimony to the great suffering and grief that HIV/AIDS causes. They reveal the courage and everyday heroism of people with HIV/AIDS, who must fight not only against a fatal disease, but against cruel treatment by family, friends, neighbours, employers and the government. They show that no class of Indians will be untouched by HIV/AIDS, that for one reason or another very many Indians are vulnerable to contracting this and other sexually-transmitted diseases. They testify that the poverty and exploitation so widespread in India and Africa make these regions particularly fertile ground for HIV/AIDS. They show how HIV/AIDS inexorably pushes families into debt and poverty. And they reveal how epidemics of HIV/AIDS take a huge toll on the economy, whether on health care, agriculture or business.

A pavement dweller

I met Jaikishan sitting on the steps outside the skin and venereal disease clinic of a government hospital in Mumbai. He is twenty-three years old, no taller than five feet and two inches, broad-shouldered but very thin, with spiky hair, wearing a lungi, faded T-shirt and rubber slippers. He is from Saurashtra in neighbouring Gujarat state. "My family owns no land," said Jaikishan. "We are of the Scheduled Castes. My father died when I was a child and my mother works as a labourer. I have a brother and sister. None of us went to school because we had to work. I can't write or read."

Since coming to Bombay four years ago, Jaikishan has worked as an unskilled labourer, lifting bricks at construction sites or freight at the railways. It is difficult to conceive of his small frame being able to lift heavy loads hour after hour. "Some days I don't get work, but on most days I can earn Rs 50 or more. I used to send money to my mother but since I've been very sick she's come to Bombay." He points to a tiny, bird-like, grey-haired woman sleeping on the pavement outside. She is barefoot, dressed in a saree that has all but lost its colours. "My cousin fetched her from the village because the doctor told me that someone would have to feed me and nurse me. Where do we sleep? I am in the hospital now. I've always slept on the pavement in Bombay so she has no place to sleep but the pavement. In January, when it was cold, she slept underneath my bed."

The impact of HIV/AIDS is most brutal on impoverished Indians like Jaikishan, who, because of our failure to reduce poverty since Independence, still make up a majority of India's people. Impoverished, illiterate, unskilled, often sick or hungry, from birth to death their lives are full of extraordinary hardships and want. Tragedy is common. The spread of HIV in India makes the likelihood of tragedy erupting in their lives even more common. And HIV/AIDS gives rise to especially harsh tragedies.

Jaikishan is sick with several infections caused by HIV/AIDS. These include chronic diarrhoea, ulcers and a crippling fungal infection, known as thrush, that carpets the throat. About eight months ago he had TB, but this was cured through treatment. "I have been here for about one month but I don't get better. This is my second time in the hospital. Last time I was less sick but had to stay here for some weeks. And then when I went back to work I couldn't work properly, I was too tired all the time, and so couldn't earn as I used to. So I don't have any money left for either of us to eat or even to buy medicines. I hear that they are meant to feed us and give us medicines for free here but nothing is free! You have to pay for the medicines, for the X-ray, to eat meat.

"I got AIDS from a woman. She was alone, a prostitute. She used to sleep near me on the pavement. I used to save her from being beaten by the police and so we started a relationship. She wouldn't take money from me, but I would feed her. She is the only person I ever had sex with. She was already sick then with a cough but what did I know? When I found out I had AIDS and was going to die, I was in terror, I couldn't sleep, I couldn't stop thinking that I would die, I cried outside the hospital all night. I then went and beat her up very badly for giving me AIDS. I'm not angry at her any more but I don't know where she's gone.

"What will we do? I don't know. My mother only earns Rs 12 when working in the village — she is an old woman — and that too not every day. And there is no one else in my family who will give us money. My brother has never given anything to my mother. What is the point of thinking about what we will do? I know I will die soon. But then what will my mother do?"

Jaikishan is one of an estimated eight to ten lakh people in Maharashtra with HIV/AIDS. Several lakhs more have already died of AIDS here. The greatest number of infected people are in Mumbai, where at the end of 1999, somewhere between three to five per cent of adults (as high as one out of every twenty) were HIV-positive. Levels of infection are as high or even higher in the state's other major towns such as Kolhapur, Nasik, Sangli, Pune, Thane and Ahmednagar. These are dangerously high levels because of the great scope for rapid increases. In the African city of Gabarone, for instance, the proportion of all adults infected rose in less than four years from six per cent — about Pune's current level — to nineteen per cent. And from Maharashtra's urban areas, HIV has for the past decade spread into the countryside. No one knows just how deeply it has penetrated. And because of seamless transport, migration and business links, the HIV/AIDS epidemic in Mumbai and Maharashtra is inextricably intertwined with that of neighbouring states such as Gujarat, Andhra Pradesh and Karnataka, all of which are now suffering from severe HIV/AIDS epidemics. Because we have better transport links and a far higher population density than Africa, experts expect that back-and-forth migration between rural and urban areas is likely to rapidly spread HIV into rural India, particularly into those areas that are the most important sources of migrant labour. This has already happened, with numerous cases of HIV/AIDS reported from, for instance, Satara district in Maharashtra and Ganjam in Orissa. As these areas comprise the heart of India's most vibrant industrial and commercial belt, the implications for our economic future are particularly worrisome. Yet, none of these state governments have begun comprehensive prevention, ranging from programmes for "higher-risk groups" to sexual health education for young people and frank awareness campaigns, that are required where HIV is so widespread.

A businessman from Mumbai

The impact of HIV/AIDS on middle class people is barely less traumatic than on the poor, even though they have more material resources to fall back on. And because the middle classes are educated, skilled or may possess assets such as businesses, the impact of HIV/AIDS on a middle class person is likely to have far-reaching repercussions on the economy.

The younger son of a prosperous farmer in Maharashtra's Sholapur district, Rajesh came to Bombay in 1982 to set up a small garment-manufacturing shop. He started out with a dozen sewing machines in East Andheri. He was just seventeen and had only finished high school. But with the boom in demand for cheap ready-made garments, he prospered. Within a decade, the single shop had multiplied into four and employed over a hundred people. Rajesh owned and ran these with a partner from Andhra Pradesh. Young, hardworking and ambitious, they were the kind of small businessmen who were essential to boosting India's economic growth and providing jobs for large numbers of people.

Beyond their partnership at work, both were partners in their almost daily visits to sex workers. Both men were married but kept their wives and children in their villages. Rajesh told me, "We wanted to have sex every day. We were crazy about sex. Of course most of the other business people we know also go to prostitutes but for the two of us it was more than a habit. With the amount of money we earned, we could pay for the best prostitutes in Mumbai. Anyway, most cost just Rs 25 or Rs 50. I'm not like Subba, who has his favourites. I never want to sleep with the same woman twice. If I realise I have had sex with her earlier, even years ago, I lose my excitement. This is why I cannot bear my wife. So I searched every time for new girls. In this city there is no shortage of women. They come from all parts of India, from every village almost, but my favourites are young Nepali girls."

He says he was handsome and muscular but today Rajesh is thin to the point of being emaciated. His six foot figure, covered by a sheet despite the heat, is lying on a wooden cot in the small flat, in a middle class Borivili housing complex, which he had bought on arriving in Bombay. He has just recovered from his third bout of tuberculosis. It was during the first bout in 1990 that he discovered that he had HIV. "This was at a government hospital in downtown Bombay. I had one or two abscesses that wouldn't heal. The hospital was dirty but the doctor was very good and explained everything about AIDS to me. I still go to that hospital because of him. He told me not to have sex with my wife or other women unless I used a condom. I've always done this, used a condom. Not because the prostitutes say anything. They are happy to earn any money, even from a man who now looks as sick as me."

After a decade of being sick — he has had bouts of several other diseases apart from TB — and paying for expensive medicines from quacks who promise to cure AIDS, Rajesh has almost no savings left. He has spent several lakh rupees on medication. He has not asked his family for money, fearing that they will visit him and discover that he has HIV/AIDS. Instead, he has sold his share in the shops to Subba, his partner, and he now works there occasionally as a supervisor. Rajesh says, "He cheated me because I was so sick and tired. But he is paying the price. Not only does he have AIDS, but so do his wife and younger children. My wife and children are not infected."

Rajesh says that he knows several young men who have HIV/AIDS. "Some own businesses like me, others are just workers or labourers. Almost no one goes back to their villages, to their families. In the village, I would bring shame to my parents. But here there are so many people sick with so many things — cholera, malaria, TB — that no one cares whether you have AIDS or some other disease. In Bombay, no one has time to bother you. Everybody thinks I have TB. I shall just die here."

A young lady in Santa Cruz

In Mumbai and other urban areas with a high proportion of adults infected, one does not need to have sex with a person with "higher-risk" behaviour to contract HIV. In fact, following the pattern in other countries, the majority of infections are now from "lower-risk" people having sex with one another. Though of course new people with higher-risk behaviours are always at greatest risk of infection. And, again following an established pattern, an ever-increasing share of infections are in young people moving into ages of increased sexual activity. This is why the Maharashtra government's unwillingness to broach broad prevention programmes, particularly sexual health education campaigns for the young, is having such fatal consequences. Gayatri Navalkar, dying at the age of twenty-nine, is one of those young people who was neither a sex worker nor ever visited a sex worker and yet contracted HIV.

When Gayatri — twenty-one years old, fresh out of college, slim, fair, doe-eyed and with long dark hair — became a sales representative with a large firm selling photocopiers, her middle class family in Mumbai's Santa Cruz area thought all their dreams had come true. Their older child, a son, was married and earning well as a junior executive with a furniture exports firm. And now their young daughter was going to earn Rs 6000 a month in a job where she would speak English and wear pretty sarees. All this amounted to success for the Navalkar family. Mr Navalkar is a senior teacher in a private secondary school and his wife a homemaker.

But five years later their dreams were in ruin. Gayatri tested positive for HIV that year, after several months of chronic diarrhoea and severe skin infections. The doctors at the private clinic threw her out even though she was covered with open sores. They told a weeping Mrs Navalkar — her husband was at school — that her daughter was a prostitute and would die for her sins. But far from being a sex worker, just a few months into her job Gayatri had been bullied, seduced and bribed into having sex by one of her most important clients, a middle-aged married man who owned a dozen photocopy stores. They continued to have an affair until he, and then Gayatri, fell sick. He was the only man whom she had ever had sex with.

There was worse to come. Everyone known to the Navalkars found out that Gayatri had HIV/AIDS. Not one neighbour from their six-storey building would visit them. The women whom Mrs Navalkar had called "Didi" gave her hate-filled looks and then turned away when she tried to approach them. At the local market, there was silence when she arrived. The crowd would move away from her as if she could infect them. A week after Gayatri had been evicted from the clinic, a letter arrived from her office saying that she had been given a month's pay as termination. Without the company's health insurance scheme they could no longer afford a private clinic, even if they could find one willing to treat her. At his school, Mr Navalkar's colleague told him that his family was a disgrace to Maharashtrian Brahmins, worse than outcastes, because of their daughter's behaviour. A few months later, their son took his wife and children and left Mumbai, never to contact his parents.

By 1999, when I met her, Gayatri was dying, a disease-ridden shadow of her attractive former self, large eyes staring out from a skeletal face, barely able to talk. The Navalkars were ruined both financially and in spirit by the costs of her medicines, by caring for her and by facing the hatred that still emanated from almost all their neighbours everyday. They sat silently while I talked with Gayatri. Their faces were exhausted but without emotion. They said they had nothing to tell me, that they were simple people with nothing to say.

A truck driver and his widow

From Mumbai, I travelled southeast to Chennai, the other city to report the first cases of HIV/AIDS in India. Though Tamil Nadu's government began with inappropriate, repressive efforts to prevent HIV, in the past five years, led by Chief Minister Karunanidhi, it has forsworn this approach and built India's most effective prevention effort. Thus, even though nearly two per cent of its adult population is infected with HIV, this is significantly lower than in Maharashtra or even in neighbouring Andhra Pradesh, where an epidemic has erupted in the past four years. Some of the essentials for effective prevention are now in place in Tamil Nadu: strong political commitment, better STD treatment services, and sexual health education programmes in schools and colleges. No less important, the state's health services are better run and equipped than all but Kerala's. And there are tentative efforts by the government to remedy the existing weaknesses in its prevention effort: make awareness campaigns less moral and more informative; establish substantive programmes for "higher-risk groups" and lessen their harassment, including men who have sex with men; and to blunt the stigma and terror around HIV/AIDS. Thus, while Tamil Nadu's situation is not optimistic — in Namakkal, over six per cent of adults are HIV-positive, the highest level in India, and levels are high in the state's other urban areas — it is now far better placed to check the epidemic than the other five states where more than one per cent of all adults are infected.

In a Chennai hospital run by a non-governmental organisation, I met Anita, the 32-year-old widow of a truck driver who had died from HIV/AIDS in November 1995. Anita was also infected and sick by the time of his death. Anita's husband was typical of other long-distance truck drivers, he probably got infected with HIV while having sex with sex workers on his trucking route. Across India, truck drivers and their helpers are amongst the occupations worst affected by HIV/AIDS. One study of seven hundred Tamil truck drivers documented that the percentage infected soared from seven out of hundred in 1992 to fifty out of hundred by 1994. Across Tamil Nadu, in fact, the percentage of truck drivers infected with HIV quadrupled from 1.5 per cent in 1995 to over six per cent just a year later. Salem, the town where Anita and her husband are from, is a centre of the trucking industry and home to many truck drivers. By the mid-1990s, about fifteen per cent of the truckers in Salem were infected with HIV.

"My husband didn't know anything about AIDS," said Anita. "He only came to know at the time of his death. He was in the hospital, the government hospital in Salem, and the doctor sent him home two days after they had told him he had AIDS saying that he was going to die. They didn't give us any advice or any medicines. They just told him to leave.

"I've studied till the eighth class. My husband had studied till the tenth. He would drive all across Tamil Nadu and to Andhra and to Karnataka. He would earn Rs 1500 or Rs 2000, I think.

"My father was a porter in a small cement factory outside Salem. My mother went for coolie work in the village. So my parents were very happy to marry me to a truck driver. And my husband also found my older brother a job as a truck driver. I don't know whether my brother has AIDS. Anyway, he doesn't send any money to my parents even though they are very poor and now look after me. My in-laws threw me and my two children out of their house when my husband died, saying I was responsible for his death. They didn't give me any money to look after them.

"The doctor here tested my children because he said they could also be infected. But they are fine. One is five years old, the other three.

"There are no problems in the community about my being sick with AIDS. On every street many other truck drivers and their wives and children have died or are sick. And we are all literate people. It is only people who don't live near Salem — like some of my relatives who live in villages — who are unwilling to come to our house or to eat here.

"I used to work in a cotton mill before I got married. But I can't go to work anymore. First I looked after my husband and since his death I've been sick all the time myself.

"My parents look after me and the children. My father is too old to work so my mother is the only one earning. She earns Rs 50 per day as a coolie, but only gets work every second day. We have a lot of debt. Once I bought Siddha medicine for AIDS from a local doctor and this cost Rs 5000. It made me even more sick. We pay Rs 300 per month in interest to the relative who gave us the money. And to come here, my father and I had to pay Rs 150 per head for the bus fare. And then we pay Rs 70 per day for food. But in the Salem hospitals, there are no doctors and no medicine.

"My parents will look after my children when I'm gone."

A sex worker and her husband

In their hut in a large slum on the city's outskirts, I talked to Jayanthi, a former sex worker, and her husband Shivakumar, who drives a scooter rickshaw. Their hut is tiny — no more than ten feet by six feet — and windowless. The narrow path outside is littered with garbage and excrement. Barefoot, frail children wander listlessly or play along the path and the densely packed huts. The slum has no toilets. It has no electricity. Half a dozen handpumps are the only source of water for the several thousand residents. The water itself is smelly and brown. Even in February, the stench and damp heat make the area oppressive.

Both Jayanthi and Shivakumar have AIDS. They have suffered several bouts of severe illness over the past five years. Jayanthi is a tiny, dark woman, who looks a decade older than her twenty years. She coughs and wheezes frequently into a man's large handkerchief. "We met in 1994 in a government hospital in Chennai," says Jayanthi. "I was in police custody in the hospital, because I was serving a sentence for being a prostitute. But because I was getting sick very often the remand home sent me to the hospital, but under police escort. Shivakumar was also sick in the hospital.

"I was born near Pondicherry in a village. My parents were agricultural labourers. My mother died when I was very young. I never had any education. When I was fourteen, one of the village women said 'Come, I will get you a job in Vellore.' But she sold me to a brothel for Rs 5000.

"There were seven other prostitutes in the brothel. They were all much older than me. I sacrificed my life in that brothel. If another prostitute had bad STDs and was in pain, I would take her place. We got STDs often. But at least we had monthly check-ups from a doctor to treat STDs and for abortions. I knew they had no doctor at other brothels. Why, in most brothels you're lucky to get fed any vegetables, so why worry about medicines.

"We would have to have sex day and night. At least ten men every day. At any time. We were supposed to get more than half of what the customer paid the madam but we were lucky to get Rs 10 out of Rs 50. She would deduct money for paying the charges for the room, for food and for working off the money she had paid for me. None of us ever complained about this. We knew better. We'd have got thrashed by the local goondas whom she used to pay.

"In 1987, after three years of this, I got arrested in a raid on the brothel. I don't know, perhaps the brothel owner had a fight with the police. Earlier, these same policemen would come many times to the brothel and have sex with us for free. In the lock-up that night the policemen beat me on my vagina with sticks. I was naked. They said it was for talking back to them.

"After that I was sentenced to five years in Vellore jail. But after two years in the jail they put me in a remand home in Chennai. The police were going to release me but as there was no parent or relative to take me — they had sent a policeman to my village but my father was working and the policeman didn't wait — the law was that I had to go forever to a remand home. They say that otherwise us women will just go back to being prostitutes. I would have liked to go home but as I couldn't the remand home was fine. What else could I have done? No one will give a job to a single woman like me, or rent me a room. And anyway what work do I know?

"The conditions in the remand home were much better than in the jail. There was no mischief going on, no rackets, because the people were very strict. If we made any mistakes, we would be caned, naked, on a bench.

"From 1989 or so I was sick all the time. At that time they took the blood of all the women in the remand home but never told us why. And then they put a whole lot of us in separate rooms. We were given special allowances of milk and eggs. The warden and other staff were very unwilling to touch us. They would serve food and water through a hole in the door. We could never understand why.

"It was only in 1994 that they told me about my having AIDS. They told me because I and some other girls were falling sick with diarrhoea, skin infections or TB. We were not told anything about what AIDS was, except that we were infected with it. We just knew it was something that we would die from. Of course we were terrified. It was only after six months that a doctor came to see us who explained what AIDS was and that we could live for some more years with good treatment.

"After meeting me in the hospital, Shivakumar married me. This was in 1995. The marriage was in the remand home. They allowed him to come to see me because he brought his mother with him. His mother was the witness at the wedding.

"We have had three children. The eldest one is four years old. The next is a bit more than one year. The youngest is just six months. She is very sick with diarrhoea and fever. All the children get sick here because of the mosquitoes and dirty water, but the little one is too weak. I think she is definitely HIV positive. All us positive people want children. Just like we want husbands or wives. We want to live. And we have children because the doctor tells us that it is not very likely that the child will be infected. I have delivered all the children at home because I know the hospitals will throw me out if they learn I have AIDS.

"I work in a charitable hospital looking after another prostitute who is dying of AIDS. I get paid by the hospital for this. And Shivakumar now drives a rickshaw. He rents it, but from this we get two to three thousand rupees a month."

Shivakumar, her husband, says, "I studied till the sixth grade. My father was a policeman in Chennai and my mother a minor actress in Tamil films. He died very early. We had lots of financial problems then, because there are five elder brothers in my family.

"I used to be a dada in my neighbourhood in Chennai. Then I went to work on a boat off Mumbai. In both places I would go with friends to sex workers. In Mumbai I went even more often because I had more money.

"I fell sick in Mumbai in 1992. So I came home to my mother's. I spent Rs 20,000 going to private hospitals but I would not get better. It was a waste, these private hospitals. The doctors were afraid of touching me even though they had gloves. They wouldn't care for me at all. And then in the last hospital I went to, the doctors suddenly told me that I was discharged and should go to a government hospital. They stood in a circle around the bed. I had a terrible wound and they said they couldn't operate. When I was leaving with my mother, the ward boy told me I had AIDS. He told me I would die very soon. The doctors had taken an AIDS test. I wanted to commit suicide but I was too weak to even kill myself.

"My mother took me to Tambaram hospital, the TB sanatorium near the airport. I weighed just twenty-three kilograms. I usually weigh more than sixty kilograms. I was there for one year. The doctor later told me I had TB, diarrhoea and a throat infection. But they made me well, even though it is a free hospital. Since then, though I have been sick often, I have only had to be admitted to Tambaram for one month. This was last year."

Jayanthi adds, "Tambaram is the one place where people with AIDS are cared for. So many prostitutes, when they get sick and get thrown out of their brothel, try to get entry to

Tambaram, even if they don't have TB. They know that there at least they will get some food and medicines. Otherwise, they will just die on the street. Once you are a prostitute, all you can do is to sell yourself. But if you look very sick, no one will pay for you however little you charge."

There are several other people sick with AIDS in their slum, said Jayanthi and Shivakumar. They know them from the city hospitals and the Tambaram sanatorium, not from living here, as all of them hide the fact that they have AIDS from others in the slum. They introduced me to two such persons.

The beauty from Chittoor

Their neighbour, Anuradha, is an astonishingly beautiful young woman, with high cheekbones, slanted brown eyes and thick black hair. She is so striking that she seems to belong on the pages of a society magazine, not in her damp, garbage-surrounded mud hut. She is only about twenty-two, but for the past two years has been increasingly sick with AIDS-related diseases, including tuberculosis. Jayanthi had told me that Anuradha was earlier a sex worker in Chennai, but is now married to a guard (who is also HIV-positive though not yet sick). Both husband and wife are from Chittoor district in Andhra Pradesh. Though both Anuradha and her husband were infected in Chennai, in Andhra Pradesh the percentage of adults infected has soared, astonishingly, in just the past four years from 0.5 per cent to well over two per cent, the most rapid increase yet in India along with Karnataka. Prevention efforts in both states are a disaster not just undertaken half-heartedly and too late, but undermined by reliance on terror and discrimination against "higher-risk groups" and people with HIV/AIDS.

Anuradha offers to make us tea. In the tiny, crowded hut, this takes half an hour. She responds to my polite questions with a "yes" or "no" in Hindi, which she speaks poorly. She is distant but gentle. Later, she tells Jayanthi in Tamil that she does not want to talk about the past or about being sick with AIDS. Jayanthi translates into broken Hindi. I say I understand and not to worry, that she has been very kind to have us as her guests, and that if I can help her in any way, at any time, she need only ask or write to me. Jayanthi translates this into Tamil. But almost as if we had said nothing, Anuradha continues in Tamil, her voice rising and her distant look replaced with anger. The beautiful woman whom countless men have lusted for disappears. In her place is a terrified child, shaking with anger at the cruelty that humans have inflicted on her. "I don't want to think about the past. I never want to think about it. I have finished with it. How will it help me to talk to you? What difference will it make if you write my story? Why should anyone care about what happened to me?" She is weeping, and though Jayanthi tries to comfort her, she turns on me angrily. "What can you do? Can you make me well? Can you give me medicines? Can you stop me from dying? You don't know anything! You don't understand anything!"

Shabnam the hijra

On the very outskirts of this large slum, on the edge of a broad open sewer thick with stinking semi-liquid refuse, is Shabnam's hut. Shabnam is a 42-year old hijra. In southern India, for reasons no one really understands, hijras do not command even the minimal respect or fear that they get in the North. In short, they are reviled and even poorer than elsewhere in India. Not surprisingly, Shabnam's hut is even more makeshift and rickety than Jayanthi's. Shabnam is dark, tall and broadly-built, though very thin, dressed in a patterned nylon saree. "I loved to dance as a child. I was always very feminine. And I would help my mother with the cooking and at home. There were no other children. My older brother died of fever when he was nine. And my younger sister died when she was very small, maybe six months old. And then my mother died when I was only about six or seven years old. My father owned a tea stall on the road outside Madurai. I used to look after him but he died when I was nineteen. There was no one left, so I went to Mumbai. I joined the hijras then. They became my friends. I lived in a rented house in Bhendi Bazaar with them. I earned most of my money through sex with men. I found out in 1992 that I was infected. I have been sick many times since then. I moved back to Chennai once I fell very sick, as I longed to be with other Tamil people. And it's cheaper here, so my savings will last longer. And they treat you better in the hospitals. In Mumbai they won't treat people with AIDS at all. When I am well, I still work as a sex worker to earn money. It's not good here, but I don't have the strength to go back to Mumbai. And anyway, most of my hijra friends there are dead or dying. Lots of Mumbai's hijras are infected. And so are many of the hijras here and in Tirupati. They formed an association in Chennai some months earlier and have got some money from the government. But it's too late for most of us."

Shabnam laughed when I asked if he told his clients to use condoms. "We have sex in a bush or a bus stand or a public urinal or even in a moving train. So who will use a condom? Who cares about sexual diseases — I and they have had many before. Who even has money to buy a condom? They fight about the Rs 10 they owe me, so you think they will pay even one rupee more for a condom! And I use my money to eat, to survive. We are not rich like you!"

A housemaid in Delhi

Travelling north to New Delhi, where almost nothing has been done in terms of HIV/AIDS prevention despite a rapidly worsening epidemic, I met Guddi, twenty-six years old, a young housemaid. Her husband died of AIDS a few months ago. She has two small children. She is a tall fair woman, neatly dressed in a blue salwar-kameez and rubber slippers. Her thick dark hair is tied in a pony-tail, secured with colourful bands. Her face is slightly made up and she wears earrings and a mangalsutra. At the NGO-run clinic where she goes for treatment for her AIDS-caused illnesses, her two young children cling to her persistently. They are also neatly dressed.

"I was married at the age of nineteen. My husband's family is from the same village and of our Jat caste. The village is in Haryana, three hours away by bus. I studied till class eight but after coming here to my husband's home I have worked at cleaning homes for people near the basti where we live. I earn Rs 1500 every month. We live in a two room pucca house. My in-laws have one room, and we have the other. My husband also studied till class eight. He was a cook in a house. And so is my mother-in-law, she cooks in the same colony in which I work. My father-in-law owns a scooter rickshaw. These are my children. The girl is six, and the boy three. Neither is infected.

"My husband slept with other women in the slum area where we live. He didn't go to prostitutes. But he slept with wives of people who were away or who didn't pay attention to what their wives were doing. I knew this, but there was nothing I could do or say.

"He had been sick for two years and then died a few months ago. He died of TB. After the first sickness he was hospitalised in the Holy Family hospital. His mother looked after him. After a few months he was again sick and this time admitted to the All-India Institute in Hauz Khas. This time my brother insisted on knowing why he wasn't recovering from the TB. We then learnt he had AIDS. He had known from the first time he was sick, and so had his parents, but none of them told me. But from the first time that he went to the hospital, he didn't have sex with me, saying that he was taking medicine for his TB.

"I was not told anything about the risks to me by the doctors in either hospital. They tested me at the second hospital. They just told me I had AIDS too. They didn't explain anything to me, just gave me the report. They are useless people anyway. They didn't even care for him. I never like going to government hospitals because of this. He was admitted twice to All-India hospital, and there they would try to not admit him and even when they did no one would touch him! But his family paid for all his medications and looked after him very well. He died at a charitable place — it is not a hospital but a place to die — near the railway station. He died of TB and other things. At this place, they taught me everything about AIDS and told me to come to this clinic for treatment. I come here once a month. If I am feeling sick, I come more often.

"I still live with my in-laws. My parents also know that I am infected and will die. So far I have not been very sick though I get tired easily and have many infections. But I try to look after myself for my children's sake. I have even put on weight. And my in-laws and parents treat me well. I go to my parents with the children sometimes. There is no discrimination of any kind, neither at my in-laws nor at my home. They all know that I am not infectious. But as I am now a widow I don't go to other people's homes. So I don't know how they would treat me.

"I worry all the time about my children. I know that my in-laws will take care of them, but they are old and then what happens?

"It would have been better for me not to have got married. I never thought that the end of my life would be like this. I would like to die quickly, not slowly, being a burden to myself and to others. I would like to die as quickly as someone who is run over by a bus."

A gay man in Daryaganj

Udai, thirty-four, is a gay man, a homosexual who acknowledges his sexual orientation. I talked to him one evening in the central park in Connaught Circle, where dozens of men congregate to search for male sexual partners, lovers or friends. "I live in Daryaganj, so it is not too far for me to come here three or four evenings a week. And it is on my way home from office. I work in a public sector firm, maintaining the computers. It's exciting work, but now I find it very tiring."

Udai prefers to speak in Hindi, but his English is quite good. "That's because I went to a good school in Jaipur. It wasn't English medium but they taught us English well. Most of the students there are from military or government families. My father is with the Rajasthan government; he is not an IAS (Indian Administrative Service) officer but with the provincial service. And my mother is a school teacher. We are Rajputs, Kshatriyas. That's why I'm so handsome. And I used to run the marathon and be a NCC (National Cadet Corps) leader."

With his sharp features, moustache, trim body and in jeans, Udai indeed attracts the interest of many of the men in the park. It is only from close up that one can tell that he is sick.

"I did my BA (Bachelor of Arts) in history and a diploma in computers in Jaipur and then moved here. I wanted to be away from my family because I always knew that I was attracted to other men. I first had sex with boys in school and then for some years with a railway ticket collector who was our tenant. Luckily, I am the youngest of two brothers and one sister, so my parents had grown tired before it came to my turn for getting married. Now of course they don't trouble me about marrying because they know how sick I've been. They know I have AIDS.

"I know many homosexual men in Delhi and Jaipur who have AIDS. And there are many more who are beginning to fall sick. I was infected a long time ago. My long-term lover is also infected. He was in the army but left because they test you all the time, and he was scared that they would tell his family. He is married and has gone back to live with his wife in Jaipur. He now runs a small transport company. We have been lovers since college. He comes here at least once a month to see me.

"Why are so many homosexual men infected? You tell me. you're the expert. Why, because none of us can talk about being homosexual. And where is the information from the government telling us that AIDS is spread by homosexual sex? You know, all these scooter-wallahs and army jawans and policemen, all of them are nearly illiterate anyway and they end up thinking that AIDS is spread only by prostitutes — by women! — because that is what the government's ads show. So gay men and even hijras are more in demand since AIDS became a problem. And some of the men think that by having anal sex you won't get AIDS so they now even have anal sex with prostitutes. And many of them think that only the passive partner can get AIDS. And many of them think that only people who look sick have AIDS. Or that only foreign men give AIDS. So none of these men here use condoms for anal sex. Only some of the boys who charge for sex — the male prostitutes — know about using condoms.

"But even us well-educated ones, what are we to do? I have used condoms since 1992. But I would put cooking oil or hair oil on the condoms to lubricate them. Half the time they would tear. Only after I got AIDS and read a lot did I learn that you cannot use oil on condoms, that it tears them. But how was I to know this? Who was there to tell me?

"I am at least lucky that I have always had a lover, even if he had to get married. At least I had his love. But the other men here, they have to be satisfied with just getting sex with one man or another. And because they can never find love and are lonely, they go about having sex with one man after another.

"There is homosexual sex everywhere — in Delhi, Jaipur, everywhere. Half the men I know have homosexual sex, even though they will never admit it. *Arre*, every type of Indian man has sex with other men, whether he is a chief minister, policeman or a scooter-wallah. It's easier than going to a prostitute and you don't have to pay. You should see how many times I have met men from my office or other government offices here or in other cruising areas. Even senior officials. We usually pretend that we have not seen each other. But sometimes we become friends.

"I've been sick for three years now. I first got sick with pneumonia. I went to this gay doctor who has a private clinic. He charges Rs 100 for consultation. But he is the only doctor who will check STDs on homosexual men. I've heard that at other places the doctors will throw you out and insult you if they find that you have STDs on your anal region or if you admit to having homosexual sex. Anyway, he told me to go for an HIV test to a counselling centre that works with gay men. They were very good there. They told me I had quite severe AIDS. I was so sick at that time that my mother took me home. My brother drove me to Jaipur in his office car. I had told her that I had AIDS but I didn't tell her that I was gay. I told her I used to go to prostitutes. But my father was so angry that he wouldn't let me into the house. She had to keep me in the store room outside. Now whenever I get very sick I go to stay in this room. My father allows me into the house to eat, but still not to stay. But I don't mind, because at least I get to see them and to be looked after. They are very good people. My father is just traditional and so he is ashamed of me, that I got AIDS. We have never spoken about it, so he has heard everything from my mother. My brothers and all don't come to the house when I'm there. They are worried that I will make their children sick.

"Whenever I'm alone all I can think about is that I have HIV. And I think about my death, that I will live for only a few more years. I used to cry a lot but now I don't. But it's only when I work or when my lover comes here — or even when I'm home with my parents — that I don't think about AIDS."

The graduate from Delhi

Rajiv is a manager with a small private sector firm in New Delhi. He has a BA in economics from a prestigious Delhi University college. A small bespectacled man in his mid-thirties, he wears a blue safari suit. His fair skin has been ravaged by recent skin infections, leaving it a pale, mottled gray. He looks exhausted. "I came to know that I had AIDS only in December 1997, but I am already very sick with several diseases," he said. "The doctor doesn't think I will live much longer. For the past two years or so I have fallen sick every fifteen days.

"My wife is also infected. She is not very sick. She has had herpes and severe skin problems. But my younger daughter is very sick with AIDS. She is only two years old. She has been sick since she was six months old. The doctor is giving her AZT for free, so for now she is okay.[8]

"What is there for me to say, for me to feel? I have cried and worried for so long now.

"Everyone in my family knows about me and my wife being sick. There were some problems initially. I live in a joint family with my brothers, and they asked me to leave the house with my family, which I had to do. Our parents are dead. But later my brothers and their wives agreed to have us back. The doctor at this hospital had explained to them that we were not a health risk to them or to their children.

"I have not told anyone in my office that I have AIDS. They would definitely sack me if they knew this. So I tell them that I am a TB patient. So far they have not suspected. But I cannot buy my medicines from the office health insurance because they would then find out what disease I have.

8 AZT or zidovudine is an antiviral drug. It is very useful for preventing HIV-transmission from an infected mother to her child during childbirth. Unfortunately, Rajiv's wife didn't get this treatment. AZT is used as a monotherapy — without other antiviral drugs — but is not effective for long, and is not recommended. Like other antivirals, it fights against the multiplication of HIV in the body and so delays the onset of disease.

"My wife began to work only after I got sick. She is working as a secretary. We are lucky because she too is educated. She has a BSc (Bachelor of Science degree). But she earns only Rs 6000 per month. I used to earn Rs 10,000 plus perks. I now earn somewhat less because I have taken a loan from the company to buy medicines. I have been able to work except for the months I have been sick in hospital. But I cannot work as fast as I used to earlier.

"We have taken about Rs 40,000 to 50,000 in loans to buy medicines and for other medical expenses for my wife, my younger daughter and me — Rs 10,000 for ayurvedic medicines, Rs 12,000 for allopathic medicines, about half of which was for AZT for my daughter; Rs 20,000 on other medical expenses, auto fares and food. We have sold our car. For two years we have lived hand-to-mouth. But I have a life insurance policy, so my family will get about two lakh rupees when I die.

"Now I know that I got HIV before I got married. I was in Mumbai in 1990 with a public sector company. A colleague at work took me to a brothel with him. And then I went once more on my own. That's it. I didn't even smoke and hardly ever drank. In 1993, I got married ..."

"I had heard about AIDS while I was in Mumbai. That it is a virus that kills you slowly. That you get if from sex. But one needs to have proper, detailed knowledge about what to do, how to protect yourself, how to have sex safely. It's not enough to know just a little bit.

"I worry most about who will look after our older daughter when my wife and I are dead. Of course, my younger daughter will die too. But who will care for my older daughter? Perhaps my wife's sister because she has two kids and so they may form a group with my daughter. My wife's sister even tells me to send her right now, but my wife and I want to keep her with us as long as we live."

Fire-fighting: Our Government's Response

If HIV is a fire and India the forest that it is roaring through, then India's politicians and bureaucrats are the reluctant firefighters who began their task half-heartedly, and then when the fire became threatening, found that they cannot match its pace. I can think of no better analogy to explain why HIV has swelled into a massive epidemic in India over the past decade-and-a-half, leaving behind limitless suffering, death and tragedy.

In the early 1990s, the government retracted from its approach of treating HIV prevention as a law-and-order problem. Its rethinking was brought on, in part, by the visible failure of this approach and by strong protests by Indian activists and lawyers against the widespread human rights abuse of sex workers, people with HIV/AIDS and other defenceless groups that the government was committing in the name of HIV/AIDS prevention. And a decisive factor was the evidence, sufficient to convince even the most sceptical officials, that HIV/AIDS was not confined to those it dismissed as "worthless" — people with higher-risk behaviours and the poor — but was affecting ever larger numbers of middle and upper class Indians, people just like them. Eventually, by 1992 or so, the Indian government took up constructive HIV prevention efforts.

Grand plans

In this second period, the government's efforts began promisingly enough. Notably, the central government took out a large loan from the World Bank for HIV/AIDS prevention, borrowing eighty-four million dollars, Rs 280 crores. The World Bank is the most influential international development organisation, along with its sister agency, the International Monetary Fund. While its policies are often immensely damaging to the interests of the average Indian, on HIV/AIDS prevention it has played a strongly positive role. As part of its agreement with the Bank, the government withdrew the draconian AIDS Prevention Bill, three years after it was first drafted by the Rajiv Gandhi government. With the money from the Bank, and grants and technical support from other international agencies, India's government now had more than sufficient financial and technical resources to undertake a comprehensive prevention effort. In fact, there was no longer any reason for India's government not to be able to prevent an epidemic of HIV/AIDS: it had ample funds, knew about the disease and how best to prevent it. Viewing these developments, in April 1992, I wrote with guarded optimism in the *Economic and Political Weekly*, "no other developing country, in Africa, or elsewhere, has been afforded such a chance. The government's decision to approach the Bank signals its willingness to accept that HIV/AIDS poses an unparalleled health and development threat. The Bank's credit will make AIDS prevention amongst the best-funded health programmes in India."

Because more than five lakh people were infected, including many with lower-risk behaviours, the prevention effort had to be far more comprehensive than in the late 1980s, when HIV was primarily concentrated amongst people with higher-risk behaviours, and that too in a few parts of the country. Now, in Maharashtra, Gujarat, Tamil Nadu and Manipur, where HIV had already spread widely, prevention efforts had to include the entire adolescent and adult population, so as to cover both people with higher and lower-risk behaviours. And because HIV was now present virtually all over India, prevention efforts with "higher-risk groups" were needed across the country. In short, quelling the further spread of HIV/AIDS now required a mammoth effort, many times broader and more complex than what was needed just half-a-decade earlier.

The central government moved to build the bureaucratic capacity needed to guide this broad prevention effort. The National AIDS Control Organisation (NACO) was established in 1992 as a semi-independent programme within the Union Ministry of Health and Family Welfare. Because it provides all the funding for state-level efforts on HIV/AIDS, through NACO the central government successfully pushed all of India's state and union territory governments into setting up state AIDS cells. NACO also formulated a slew of policies relating to different aspects of HIV prevention and worked with the state AIDS cells on initiating programmes based on these policies. Aided and prodded by NACO, in these early years some state governments took substantial action, particularly Tamil Nadu, Maharashtra and Kerala.

NACO and the state AIDS cells made plans for a huge range of interventions, and began to implement some of them.

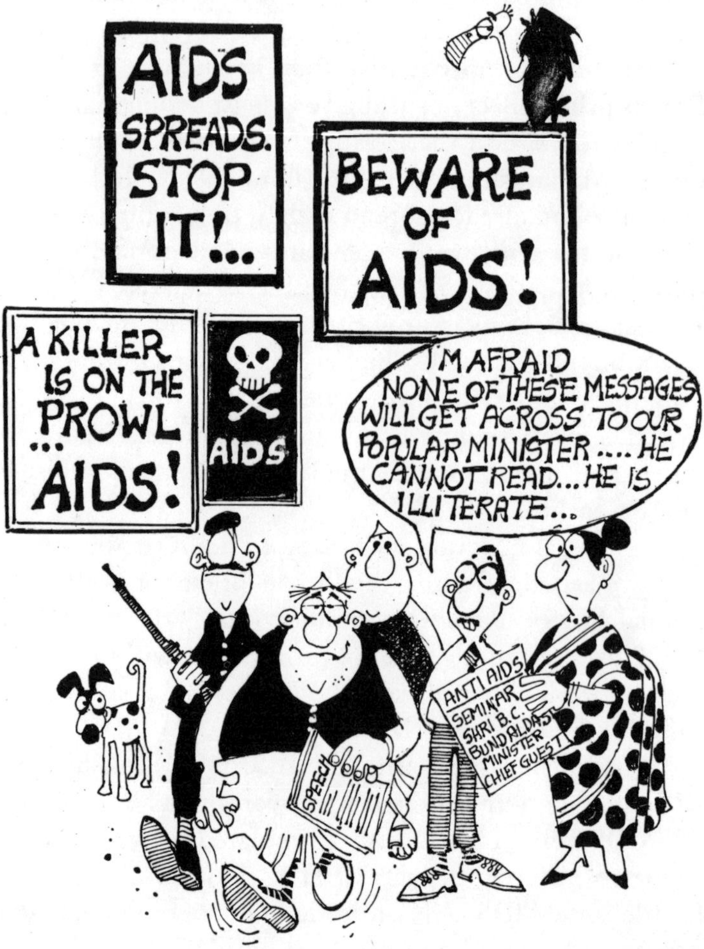
AIDS
SPREADS.
STOP
IT!...
BEWARE
OF
AIDS!
A KILLER
IS ON THE
PROWL
...
AIDS!
AIDS
I'M AFRAID
NONE OF THESE MESSAGES
WILL GET ACROSS TO OUR
POPULAR MINISTER .... HE
CANNOT READ... HE IS
ILLITERATE...
ANTI AIDS
SEMINAR
SHRI B.C.
BUNDALDAS
MINISTER
CHIEF GUEST
SPEECH

Both through the central Information and Broadcasting Ministry and through state government efforts, general HIV/AIDS awareness campaigns were begun, using the print, radio and television media. Workshops were held to sensitise key media people, including commercial film makers. A "Universities Talk AIDS" programme was launched in over two hundred colleges, with the goal being to cover all major universities and government senior secondary schools. Advocacy meetings were undertaken with a wide range of opinion leaders and policy makers, corporate and industrial leaders, and private sector doctors and nurses.

Plans were made to improve the government's STD clinics through developing training materials and courses, improving the miserable supply of drugs and basic laboratory equipment, and formulating detailed treatment guidelines. An awareness campaign was planned to encourage people to seek treatment for their STDs. Government health functionaries at all levels, even in the most basic clinics, were to be trained to recognise and treat STDs by broad symptoms. The training was to emphasise the importance of not discriminating against those with STDs. And as the majority of STD patients use private sector doctors or health practitioners, NACO worked with the Indian Medical Association, a major grouping of doctors, to develop a training programme for private practitioners in STD treatment.

To track trends in the spread of HIV, a serosurveillance network was established in major urban areas, covering most of the states and union territories. And to better understand sexual practices, a risk-behaviour survey was begun of sixty-five cities, mapping the populations engaged in risky behaviours and assessing how non-governmental organisations (NGOs) could best assist these groups.

A large share of the funds for HIV/AIDS prevention was earmarked for cleaning up the blood supply. Despite the large amount of money spent from 1986 to 1991, India's blood supply was still unsafe. Many private and government blood banks were registered with the Drug Controller but were not licensed. There were numerous clandestine blood banks, no one knew how many. About one-third of the blood supply still came from professional "donors" who were paid for their blood by commercial blood centers. To curtail the risks of blood-borne HIV infection, routine screening of all blood and blood products was essential. The use of professional blood donors had to be ended. The supply of blood had to come from voluntary, unpaid donations from the general public, as is the pattern in richer countries. And health staff needed to be trained to avoid unnecessary blood transfusions, a very common practice in India.

Guidelines for the participation of NGOs were developed, and funds released to the states for funding NGOs. Soon, scores of NGOs were working on HIV/AIDS prevention. Several of these NGOs, with funding from the government or from international donors, began programmes to reach sex workers, truck drivers, migrant workers, professional blood donors, drug users and other high-risk groups. And to find ways of reducing human rights abuses related to HIV/AIDS, a sub-committee on social, legal and ethical issues was set up within NACO.

In mid-1994, I was part of a World Bank team reviewing the government's performance on HIV/AIDS. I had joined the Bank's health and nutrition department in early 1993, and left at the end of 1994, returning to Delhi to write a book on poverty. I can recall how at that time, viewing all that the central government and some state governments had achieved, for the first time I felt optimistic that India would be spared a devastating epidemic.

Too little too late

My optimism evaporated rapidly. From 1995 to 1997, while doing research for the poverty book in Uttar Pradesh and Mumbai, I realised that the government's commitment had faltered dangerously when it came to implementing these fine plans, especially the sexuality-related programmes that form the core of effective HIV/AIDS prevention. Tragically, the government's efforts have never recovered momentum. This is true of NACO itself, as well as virtually every state programme apart from Tamil Nadu's. Some action has been taken, but always half-heartedly and too little and too late to keep ahead of the epidemic's wild-fire spread. And as the epidemic grows, its control requires not just more money, but more radical and forthright actions, which the government continually fails to deliver. The net result is that India's government continues to fall ever further behind in the deadly race against the epidemic.

Ironically, the growing chasm between the epidemic's growth and the official response has been masked because there is now the appearance of so much activity related to HIV/AIDS: NACO itself, state AIDS cells with ample budgets, innumerable newspaper and research articles, huge media campaigns, experts and conferences galore, fund-raising events by celebrities, HIV/AIDS telephone hot-lines in the big cities, innumerable teams from international donors and agencies, hundreds of NGOs, much data, World AIDS Day campaigns...and so on. Looking at all this, anyone would assume that HIV/AIDS was being beaten. Unfortunately, all this activity adds up to too little in terms of impact. This is not to deride the great efforts and commitment of the people working on HIV/AIDS in the government and outside. The result is that HIV continues to spread across India with juggernaut-like force. Apart from the forty to fifty lakh Indians already infected, four thousand or more are infected every day, a pace so relentless that the number of people infected doubles within eighteen to twenty-four months. This is the dangerous rut where we remain stuck today.

The government's failure on HIV/AIDS prevention is rooted in continued denial by most of our political and bureaucratic leaders that India can ever suffer from a full-blown epidemic of HIV/AIDS. The denial is of course deeply perplexing given the fifty lakh Indians infected, the twenty to twenty-five lakhs dead, and the three to five per cent of adults infected in over half-a-dozen urban areas. Unfortunately, one of the many twists of HIV/AIDS is that most deaths caused by it are ascribed to the common infections like TB and diarrhoea that kill these adults. How many times have I cringed inwardly on hearing the question, "Oh, if so many people are dying of AIDS, why don't we notice?" If only HIV/AIDS was as visible as smallpox! It is only now that doctors in cities like Mumbai, Pune and Chennai, where tens of thousands of people have died from AIDS, are familiar with the clinical features of the disease, but doctors elsewhere in India still lack this experience. The upshot is that until today only a small number of officials, typically those working on HIV/AIDS prevention or other health issues, have realised just how disastrous the situation is in India. Others, particularly senior politicians, continue to deny — despite the best advice — that the virus has spread in epidemic proportions in India and that prevention must take place now, not wait until crores of people are dead.

Unfortunately, without visible political leadership even large budgets and formal programmes are inadequate to check HIV/AIDS. In the handful of developing countries that have succeeded in slowing their epidemics — Thailand, Uganda and Senegal — their political heads (for instance, President Museveni of Uganda and Prime Minister Panyarachun of Thailand) personally led the national HIV/AIDS campaigns. They promoted condom use, sex education and STD treatment. They put an end to the misguided attempts to forcibly test or quarantine those suspected of higher-risk behaviours. They ensured that the rights of people with HIV/AIDS would be protected. They urged an open, nationwide discussion of sexual behaviours and of how these needed to change because of HIV/AIDS. Without doubt the greatest benefit of their leadership was that it diminished the stigma attached to HIV/AIDS. Prevention programmes with "higher-risk groups" began to work, as people from these groups and those already infected knew that their rights would be protected. HIV/AIDS became a respectable, legitimate problem, just like any other, rather than a cause of shame and discrimination. There was open and freer discussion of sexual issues and HIV/AIDS. And when it turned into a legitimate mainstream problem, other leaders — whether from military, academic, media, corporate, trade union, community and even religious groups — felt encouraged to undertake constructive work in their fields. Consequently, in these countries the governments' prevention efforts gradually grew into something approaching a public mass movement and the number of new infections began to fall.

A commitment problem

But in India, so far, there has been a saddening lack of top-level political commitment to HIV/AIDS prevention. Between

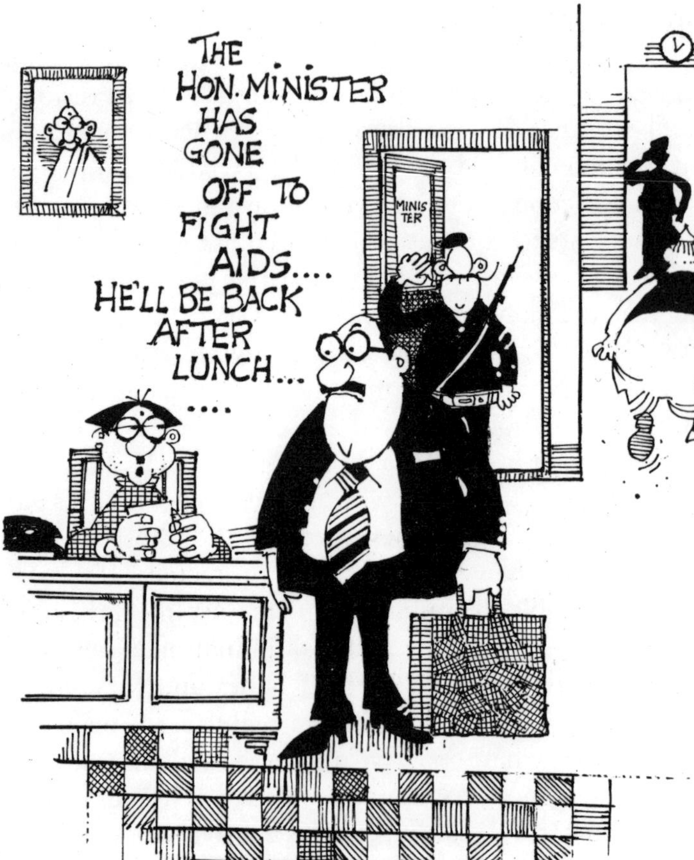
THE HON. MINISTER HAS GONE OFF TO FIGHT AIDS.... HE'LL BE BACK AFTER LUNCH... ....
MINIS TER
SPEECH

1992 and end-1999, the four prime ministers and two presidents of this period made only a handful of statements about the threat posed by HIV/AIDS. In all, they probably did not comment on this issue on more than a dozen separate occasions. Anyhow, their statements were usually so guarded and woolly that the sexual issues at the heart of HIV transmission were hidden. (In 1998, Prime Minister Vajpayee commendably broke this silence about sex, urging that young people be taught about "sexual and reproductive health".) And altogether, these leaders met less than a dozen times with people with HIV/AIDS. Then too they chose to meet such "innocent victims" as children and haemophiliacs. They shunned the lakhs of infected sex workers, and the even larger number of infected men who were their clients, and the lakhs of men infected by having sex with other men, and the tens of thousands of infected drug users. The lack of political commitment was so strong that though a visionary National AIDS Prevention and Control Policy was written in 1997 it was only approved by the Cabinet two years later.[1]

The record of chief ministers of state and union territory governments is even more depressing. As health is a state subject, only leadership by chief ministers can ensure that HIV/AIDS prevention gets top political priority. But our chief ministers — whether with the BJP, Congress, Left Front, or from the regional parties — have been virtually silent on HIV/AIDS. This is so even in such badly affected states as

1 Anyhow, national policies are barely worth the paper they are printed on as they are not legally enforceable. Revealingly, a progressive national policy on HIV-testing was passed five years ago, but few state-level officials even know about it, let alone adhere to it. The chances of the Prevention and Control Policy actually making a difference would increase were it passed by Parliament as a law. Unfortunately, there are still no plans to do so.

Maharashtra, Andhra Pradesh, Karnataka, Manipur and Delhi. Leadership in these states is so lacking that in 1999 both the Karnataka and Maharashtra assemblies considered bills that would have allowed mandatory testing, quarantine and other coercive policies, an approach that should have been put to rest a decade ago. The sole exception to this sorry pattern is Chief Minister Karunanidhi of Tamil Nadu, who since 1997 has had the foresight to encourage prevention and the political courage to meet people with HIV/AIDS. His backing has been crucial to Tamil Nadu building India's most effective HIV-prevention effort, though even this could be greatly improved.

How about union ministers, members of parliament and top bureaucrats? With a few notable exceptions, their record on HIV/AIDS is miserable. On several occasions, the union health ministers of this period have publicly disputed the scale of the HIV/AIDS problem in India, insisting that the situation was not as bad as reported by international organisations. Thus, in 1997, Saleem Shervani accused the World Health Organisation of exaggerating how badly India was affected. Worse, some union ministers have actively harmed HIV/AIDS prevention efforts. As communication and information minister, Sushma Swaraj banned a popular FM radio programme on safe sex, saying that Indians should be educated on values, not on sexuality. Only a few ministers have had the foresight and political courage to champion HIV/AIDS. Notably, the Communist Party of India's Indrajit Gupta, while home minister, participated in the National Convention of Sex Workers of India, in November 1997, which brought together several thousand male, female and hijra sex workers in Calcutta, demanding recognition of sex work as an occupation and workers' rights. Our MPs? They have been so indifferent that only a dozen attended a meeting on HIV/AIDS called by Prime

Minister Vajpayee in December 1998. Our most senior bureaucrats outside the ministry of health? Silent!

The fallout

What has the appalling lack of commitment by the country's top political and policy-making leadership led to?

- First, it has meant that India's political establishment, comprised of those who come below these top leaders, whether in New Delhi or in state capitals, have no reason to give HIV/AIDS prevention much importance.
- Second, it has meant that NACO has become increasingly sidelined within the central government. Its ability to push for national action or to assist the states has rapidly dwindled.

Tellingly, it took the government nearly five years to bring the government-manufactured Nirodh condoms — which were non-lubricated and frequently tore during use — up to acceptable safety standards. There is no doubt that in the interim many people contracted HIV despite faithfully following the government's advice to use condoms. And despite spending crores on this task, by late 1996 the government had so visibly failed to improve regulation of blood supplies that the Supreme Court was driven to order that blood banks that failed to test for HIV would be closed down.[2] A year later,

2 By 1994, eight years into India's epidemic, the best estimates suggested that only half of India's blood supply was being screened. Even large urban blood banks were routinely violating HIV-screening regulations. For instance, in 1995, Mumbai's premier blood bank, operated by the Bombay branch of the Indian Red Cross Society, was shut down by authorities after it was proved that HIV-testing equipment was often broken, lab technicians were selling contaminated blood earmarked for disposal, and dozens of children had contracted HIV from blood supplied by it.

in desperation the court outlawed the practice of selling blood. Despite all this, the problem of unsafe blood persists. As this is the one aspect of HIV prevention most amenable to a technical solution, the government's poor performance on this front says a lot about how poorly it must be tackling aspects of prevention centred on people.

Third, with no leadership from either top central government figures or their own state-level leaders, staff at the state AIDS cells have neither pressure to perform nor the influence to push others. So even uncontroversial but important prevention efforts — for instance, public awareness campaigns, STD services or blood safety — have not been implemented well or on the scale needed by the state AIDS cells. These efforts have been undertaken in a bureaucratic manner, marked by inefficiency and uninspired thinking. In many states, including Delhi, the heads of the AIDS cell have been changed several times a year.

Awareness campaigns have been so morally conservative that they fail to convey the basic issues involved in sexual transmission of HIV/AIDS, or worsen the stereotyping and terror about the disease. The chasm between the fine plans laid in the early 1990s and reality is so vast that as late as end-1999, STD treatment services had not been noticeably improved anywhere in India apart from Tamil Nadu. Even in Delhi, right under NACO's nose, prevention amounts to little more than billboards even today. Little prevention work has been done with sex workers or other particularly vulnerable groups, only two of the city's seven voluntary HIV-testing centres provide counselling. Doctors still refuse to treat people with HIV/AIDS, and supplies needed to maintain universal precautions aren't available in public hospitals, even gloves and cotton wool are often missing. Overall, the performance of most state AIDS cells has been so poor that they have regularly failed to spend funds that have been allocated to them by the central government.

Even more damaging, the lack of top-level leadership has meant that neither the central nor most state governments have been committed to the task of broaching the inherently more controversial sexuality-related programmes that are essential to HIV/AIDS prevention. Sexual health education programmes for youth have been a tragic victim of this lack of commitment. Research from many settings has shown that comprehensive sexual health education in schools promotes safer sex while actually decreasing sexual activity amongst young people. It is important to begin sexual health education early, as adolescents who are not yet sexually active and get information about HIV/AIDS delay their first sexual experiences and have fewer sexual partners than students who get information after they have begun sex.

By the mid-1990s, the National Council of Education Research and Training had belatedly come around to advocating that meaningful sexual health education programmes be made part of the curriculum of secondary schools. But education is a state subject, and no state apart from Tamil Nadu has pressed ahead with sexual health education in schools. To the contrary. In the mid-1990s, caving in to protests from conservative groups, the Maharashtra government banned AIDS education in public schools, despite having the worst epidemic of any Indian state. At the end of 1999, Gujarat's officials were still arguing over whether to allow sex education in schools. The situation is just as bad at college level. There are no formal sexual health or HIV/AIDS education programmes for college students. And the impact of the well-planned Universities Talk AIDS Progamme has been undermined by half-hearted implementation.

- Equally disastrous are the programmes needed by people with higher-risk sexual behaviours. They require programmes on HIV/AIDS and STD awareness, treatment for STDs, condom promotion, and voluntary counselling and anonymous testing. (If they inject drugs, they also need other kinds of support.)

These programmes deserve top priority, to prevent further infections, to provide those infected with early preventive care for illnesses, and to counsel them about safer sex so that others are not infected. But until today only a small percentage of those at higher risk of contracting HIV are being reached by appropriate prevention programmes. No less disastrous, their persecution by government officials and the police persists. This is true of the entire gamut of people with higher-risk sexual behaviours. Consequently, the number of infections amongst sex workers and every other "higher-risk group" continues to climb in almost every part of India. This is so even in Tamil Nadu, which has built the country's best overall prevention effort. The sole exception to this depressing rule is Calcutta, where infection rates amongst sex workers have been held at a low level. Calcutta's success, exemplified by a project in the Sonagachi "red light" area, stems from the fact that sex workers have unionised and battled the causes of their vulnerability. Particularly in Sonagachi, sex workers now have better health care and STD treatment services, force customers to use condoms, fight against police harassment, and have begun schools for their children and savings schemes for themselves.

🎗 Amongst the "higher-risk groups," the gap between need and action is widest with regard to men who have sex with men. This is true across India. Though NACO has belatedly accepted that sex between men is indeed an important cause of the country's epidemic, in practice almost every central or state-level official in charge denies the need to begin prevention efforts for such men. Given this persisting denial, there are no government programmes and only about half-a-dozen NGO programmes on promoting safe sex amongst these many lakhs of men. Nor has NACO pushed with any evident result to get jail or remand home authorities to agree to undertake HIV/AIDS prevention with inmates. Without doubt, these failures have led thousands of male undertrials and convicts in jails and boys in remand homes to contract HIV in these years.

The blame game

Anyhow, even the existing NGO and government programmes with "higher-risk groups" have rarely had much impact. This is because the central and state governments have failed to reduce the terrible discrimination and persecution faced by these groups and by people with HIV/AIDS. This abuse drives underground people with HIV/AIDS or those concerned that they are infected, making prevention impossible. Ironically, though it has been nearly a decade since the central government formally repudiated coercive HIV/AIDS prevention policies, such abuse continues across India (with West Bengal an exception so far) on the orders of state government, judicial and police authorities. In fact, the abuse is now so legion as to defy cataloguing. Unsurprisingly, the stigma, fear and discrimination around HIV/AIDS that grew out of the repressive prevention policies of the1980s have worsened, as is testified to by the unrelieved terror gripping the people whose stories were told in the previous chapter.

Until today sex workers are arrested and forcibly tested for HIV; those found to be positive are quarantined. They, and often men who have sex with men, are harassed, blackmailed and forced into sex by lower-level policemen. Drug users are imprisoned. In this atmosphere of blame, each year some new group is accused of spreading HIV/AIDS; truck drivers are the latest scapegoat. The confidentiality of people testing positive for HIV is regularly breached by doctors or by other hospital staff. On learning that their patients have HIV/AIDS, doctors in both public and private hospitals simply deny them care and throw them out. Without the counselling that would have helped them to cope with their terrors, many people have committed suicide. In hundreds of documented cases, these breaches of confidentiality and resulting discrimination have led to people being thrown out of their jobs (including those with the armed forces), homes and neighbourhoods. HIV tests are now demanded as part of pre-employment medical tests by many employers and those testing positive are denied employment. In 1999, the Indian Navy declared that it would not re-engage or promote HIV-positive staff.

Such abuse is particularly common in Maharashtra, even though it was the first Indian state to begin work on HIV/AIDS prevention and so has had ample time to learn that coercion does not work. Its politicians, judges, bureaucrats and police continue to victimise people from "higher-risk groups" or those with HIV/AIDS. In 1994, the Maharashtra government drafted and fought bitterly to pass a bill that would have allowed them to brand HIV-positive sex workers with indelible ink. In 1996, the Mumbai High Court, on its own initiative, ordered the arrest of 400-odd sex workers and their mandatory screening for HIV.[3] They were kept in custody for over a year, during which time seven died. Those found to be positive were deported to their own states, or, in the case of Nepalese women, back to Nepal. In end-1997 a government order required all boarding homes for homeless girls to conduct mandatory tests for HIV on girls within forty-eight hours of their arrival, and to quarantine those found positive.

But the thinking of Maharashtra's judiciary, government and police has a powerful influence across India. In 1997, in Haryana's Chochi village, the entire adult population was forcibly tested for HIV on the orders of the district administration, on the grounds that a "quack" physician may have infected them by using unsterilised hypodermic needles. Raids and forcible testing of sex workers are common everywhere. The national Supreme Court, in a judgement concerning Agra's sex workers, decided that they could be tested for HIV regardless of their consent. And at the end of 1998, the Supreme Court ruled that people with HIV or AIDS could not marry, "as the marriage would have the effect of spreading the infection of his own disease, which is obviously dangerous to life, to the woman he marries." This ruling is particularly ill-informed. Its simplistic and coercive approach is no different to the government's strong-arm methods in the 1986-1991 period. For precisely the same reasons it is destined

3 The Mumbai High Court has, however, made some progressive rulings on HIV/AIDS. In 1997, it established that discrimination against employees who are HIV-positive is not permissible unless the employee poses risk of transmission to colleagues or is unable to fulfill job requirements. This ruling has helped curtail dismissals of employees with HIV/AIDS by both public and private sector employers.

to fail. It perpetuates the myth that people with HIV/AIDS are criminals who cannot be trusted. By compelling doctors and medical staff to disclose the HIV status of their patients, it forces people concerned about their HIV status to stay away from testing and other medical services, when greater use of these services is critical to prevention. (Tellingly, the National AIDS Prevention and Control Policy, approved by the Cabinet some months later, does not favour the Supreme Court's approach, preferring voluntary disclosure by the infected party.) None of this is to deny that there are now several documented instances of women and girls being married off to men who know they are HIV-positive and purposely hide this from their future wives. But the Supreme Court could have achieved its creditable concern about this abuse by instructing the central and state governments to begin public campaigns encouraging voluntary pre-marriage tests for HIV and other STDs. Families of the betrothed would have asked each other for these certificates. They would also become more aware and knowledgeable about STDs and HIV/AIDS. And parents would have been forced to discuss sexuality, STDs and HIV/AIDS with their children.

The central government must bear a great part of the blame for the unabated abuses related to HIV/AIDS. By not passing a comprehensive law that would cover the entire gamut of human rights issues related to HIV/AIDS in India, it has left these issues open to the vagaries of state governments and judiciaries. Consequently, there are no checks on coercion or discrimination by state governments, the judiciary, police, medical staff or employers. And when such abuse is challenged in court, India's judges have rarely ruled in an informed and progressive manner.

The central government's weak commitment to protecting those infected or those most vulnerable to HIV/AIDS is evident in many other areas, with equally disastrous results. NACO has made little progress in ensuring that medical staff in government institutions (let alone those in the private sector), do not deny care to those with HIV/AIDS. Until today NACO has not included people with HIV/AIDS or those from higher-risk groups in policy-making on HIV/AIDS. With this, NACO forgoes learning from their knowledge about HIV/AIDS. No less important, it also misses a singular chance to improve their visibility and status and so reduce the discrimination they suffer.[4] And NACO still refuses to agree that anonymous testing — where people who come for tests are given only a number and do not reveal their names — is preferable to the current practice of so-called "confidential" testing, in which health staff know the patient's name and routinely disclose the identity of those who are infected to the media or to others. Only a handful of progressive NGOs provide anonymous testing, such as the Naz Foundation in Delhi and YRG Care in Chennai. Given people's very real fear that their identities will be disclosed and that they have nothing to gain, few make use of the government's expanded HIV-testing facilities. This is a great opportunity going to waste. Voluntary testing and follow-up counselling are very effective in getting both infected and uninfected people to reduce risky behaviours. People who learn early that they are infected can begin inexpensive preventive treatment to avoid tuberculosis and

4 There are now plans to include people with HIV/AIDS and those from "higher-risk groups" in state AIDS societies. But, unfortunately, they are likely to only have token representation. To make this exercise more than mere window-dressing, they need to be full and equal partners, with the ability to influence policies and to shape implementation. But such partnerships can never emerge if people fear harassment or stigmatisation.

several other diseases. And therapy of infected mothers with AZT or other antiviral drugs improves the chances that their newborns will not be infected.

Tragically, in the years ahead, there is no reason to expect that the central and state governments will do any better on HIV/AIDS prevention than they have done in the past decade. We should only expect more of the same: at the central level, visionary plans that are undermined by denial and inadequate political commitment; and at the state level, shoddy implementation, recourse to coercive policies, and a persisting climate of fear and terror. One can expect nothing better than this bleak outcome even though the Indian government has taken out a second and even larger World Bank loan for HIV/AIDS prevention. The loan makes a total of 191 million dollars — nearly Rs 800 crores — available to the government. Counting assistance from other donors and agencies, the government has nearly 300 million dollars on hand for HIV/AIDS control. This much money is sufficient to mount an effective effort against HIV/AIDS, even with fifty lakh Indians infected. But money can do precious little to combat the denial and indifference that continues to grip India's political and bureaucratic leaders and, relatedly, their refusal to address sexual issues honestly.[5] So the crores from this loan, like those from the first loan, will again be frittered away. Some of it will certainly fund a few effective efforts, but the bulk will go to routine programmes with low impact or to completely worthless things. All this activity and huge expenditure will

5 Unfortunately, the World Bank rushed to give the second loan without a comprehensive prior review of why the first loan had done so poorly. By doing this, it foreclosed a rare chance for engaging the Indian public in a discussion about HIV/AIDS and why prevention was failing, and very importantly, for leveraging policy changes in the government.

help save only a tiny percentage of people who would have otherwise ended up contracting HIV. Of course, this is better than no one being saved at all. Given our huge population, even a small percentage of people saved from HIV totals up to lakhs of people.

But overall, HIV will continue to spread relentlessly across India, with ever larger numbers of people infected each year. The best estimates show that the number of Indians infected with HIV is growing so rapidly as to double every eighteen to twenty-four months. Hence, the World Bank anticipates that without successful prevention, by 2005 about five per cent of our adult population — 3.5 to four crore people — will have contracted HIV. If current trends persist, this number could easily cross ten crores in another couple of years. Whatever the exact numbers, within the next decade several crore Indians are likely to be sick and dying of HIV/AIDS and even larger numbers will be infected. This *Kali Yug*, this apocalypse, has already begun to engulf us.

Charred Lands: Africa's Present, India's Future?

To understand just how horrific this future is, come with me to the African countries that have been living out what we are almost certain to suffer in the years just ahead. We Indians have much to learn from Africa about HIV/AIDS, both good and bad. So read slowly.

Neither words nor numbers can describe the horror that HIV/AIDS has created in Africa. The sickness and death inflicted on crores of people. The grief inflicted on their surviving children, relatives and friends. The ravaging of families and communities. The worsened poverty, foregone economic growth and reversed development. The even greater number of deaths and more severe losses that inevitably lie ahead. Take the total of the bombs, deaths and agony of the two world wars, locate them in a single continent, and even that carnage would be dwarfed by that being wrought in

Africa by HIV/AIDS. Destruction on this scale defies description, defies comprehension.

I first visited Africa in 1991. This was for a United Nations workshop on HIV/AIDS held in Kenya which brought together people from almost every continent. By then, in the worst-affected African countries, all to the south of the Sahara desert, over seventy-five lakh adults and children had contracted HIV and lakhs had already died. The epidemic's disastrous impact on agriculture, health care, business and overall development prospects was already evident and was ceaselessly intensifying. Many of the Africans at that workshop had turned to working on HIV/AIDS because the disease had infected or killed their lovers, siblings, parents, friends. Some were infected or sick themselves. They all bore a sorrow as well as a passion about fighting this disease that was lacking in those of us from Asia or elsewhere where HIV had yet to hit with full force. They also bore a despair, a despair about whether their governments would ever act strongly before the epidemic became uncontrollable in their countries.

Already shaken by the tragedies I had seen just months earlier on my first HIV/AIDS-related journey across India, in the weeks that I spent at the workshop I ingested some of their sorrow and some of their passion. But most, I ingested their despair about governments anywhere stemming HIV/AIDS in time. On leaving the workshop I toured, on work, other parts of Kenya, the former French Congo and Malawi, but I saw nothing to ease my pessimism. In each the number of people getting infected was soaring relentlessly. Much like in India, there was sex and STDs aplenty, the tinderbox for HIV. Health services were even worse than in India, partly a result of the economic and foreign debt crisis that has crippled these countries since the 1980s. In Malawi's urban areas nearly every fifth adult was infected, yet reliable condoms were still barely available. And like India's leaders and decision-makers, the leaders of these countries insisted that their society's morals were better than those of their neighbours, or that HIV was a disease of only the deviant and the poor. In other words, that their countries would never suffer from HIV/AIDS epidemics.

In the next three years, I went back several times to Africa, working on the World Bank's health and HIV/AIDS projects in Kenya and Uganda. Each time, my pessimism deepened, not just about the situation in Africa but by extension also about India. In an ever-increasing number of African countries, the number of people getting infected was multiplying at mind-boggling speed. But, almost without exception, none of their governments was acting in any real sense, or their efforts lagged far behind what was needed. By the time of my last trip, in mid-1994, one crore Africans had HIV/AIDS. In Kampala, Uganda's capital, nearly every third adult was infected. As Kenya's government had done virtually nothing in terms of prevention, fifteen per cent of adults were infected in urban areas, double the 1990 level.

In the subsequent years the despair of my African colleagues at that Kenya workshop has been proved correct. In much of Africa HIV/AIDS is now simply a fire out of control. Because governments have not acted sufficiently early (or at all) and because the snowballing epidemic has far outstripped their resources, in about half-a-dozen African countries twenty-five to thirty-three per cent of all adults are now infected with HIV, every fourth or even third adult. In many others, between five and fifteen per cent of the adults are infected. In several cities, every second adult is infected. Imagine walking on a city street and realising that every other adult you see — including those barely out of their teens — will die in a matter of years from HIV/AIDS. The sharpest increases in the past decade have been in populous South Africa and wealthy Botswana, where up to one in three adults is infected in urban areas. Only a handful of African countries have done relatively well in combating HIV — Senegal and more recently, Uganda. Altogether, about 2.3 crore Africans are infected with HIV and will die within a few years: 1.2 crore women, one crore men and ten lakh children.

And another 1.4 crore have already died. In some countries, entire generations have been wiped out. Many villages are no more than ghost communities, peopled only by the dying, the very old and the very young. Yet the death toll increases each year. In 1998 alone, about eighteen lakh Africans were killed by AIDS. HIV/AIDS is not only Africa's worst killer-disease, it has probably killed more Africans than all of that continent's bloody wars in the past fifty years.[1]

As its toll is mainly on adults in their sexually active years, AIDS is now the primary cause of adult deaths in much of Africa. In some areas, it has more than doubled the adult death rate. Most of those dying are in the prime of their

1 Apart from the 2.3 crore Africans with HIV, another one crore people are infected worldwide. Of these, about forty lakhs are in India; fifteen lakhs in Thailand and other Southeast Asian countries; five to ten lakhs in China (and other East Asian nations); 2.2 lakhs in North Africa and the Middle East; 3.5 lakhs in Eastern Europe and Central Asia; seventeen lakhs in Latin America and the Caribbean; and fifteen lakhs in the industrialised countries. HIV/AIDS has made deep inroads into new regions in the 1990s. Levels of infection are now as high in some southern African countries as in East and Central Africa, where the epidemic first took hold; in Asia, more than sixty lakh people are infected; in the former Soviet Union, HIV rates have doubled in the past two years; and the countries of the Caribbean basin have some of the worst HIV epidemics outside Africa.

life — from the early twenties to the mid-fifties — who would otherwise have lived and worked for many years more. Through infections transmitted from mother to child, the effect on infant and child mortality is equally devastating. About twenty-five lakh African babies have been born with HIV, and most have already died from it. Driven by these increases in both adult and child mortality, life expectancy in fifteen African nations is now eleven years shorter than it would have been had HIV/AIDS never appeared. In the worst-hit countries like Botswana, Zimbabwe and Zambia, life expectancy has fallen by thirty years or so.

The epidemic has overwhelmed health care systems in most African countries. As in India, these countries' public health systems were almost always under-staffed, under-financed and poorly run. Not surprisingly, hospitals, clinics and medical personnel have been unable to cope with the huge number of people suffering from HIV/AIDS. In many African countries, HIV/AIDS patients occupy fifty to eighty per cent of the beds in some hospitals, displacing patients suffering from other diseases. The costs of treating them are also higher than for other patients, worsening the budgetary strains. The drain on government health budgets leaves little for basic health care needs, including immunisations and treatment for other illnesses. As a consequence, other diseases are flourishing. TB, with its close interaction with HIV, is particularly rampant. In several countries, the number of TB cases has doubled or trebled from already very high levels. These stresses on already crumbling health systems are further exacerbated because thousands of Africa's scarce doctors and nurses have themselves died of HIV/AIDS.

Because the vast majority of those who contract HIV are adults — and hence typically parents and breadwinners — their sickness and eventual death typically destroys whatever material security the family possessed. The loss of a critical breadwinner is devastating, pushing middle class families into poverty and the poor into deeper poverty. The family's finances first suffer from the costs of medicines, care and lost work-days. Like most Indians, the average African can barely afford medicines, even less so when they are too sick with HIV/AIDS to work. They need someone to care for them, and consequently both the sick person and their care-givers miss work. Children drop out of school to care for their parents or to till their farms. Many people with HIV/AIDS lose their jobs, often because of discrimination.

The impact on family structures is equally devastating. In a tragic reversal of roles, the elderly bury their adult children, often all their children. They not only lose the support of those who should have provided for them in their old age, but must typically also care for their grandchildren. Often, elderly African grandparents are found caring for a dozen grandchildren. But amongst the most devastated and numerous survivors are orphaned children. Over one crore African children — equal to Delhi's entire population — have lost either one or both parents. Some of them are being looked after by relatives, usually by grandparents. Others are in orphanages. The vast majority are on the street. These young children, many just four or five years old, beg, steal and turn to prostitution to survive.

Cumulatively, the illness and death of these thousands and lakhs of working-age and productive adults has undermined communities, industries, whole sectors of the economy and society at large. The true costs of the epidemic in Africa are almost incalculable and are only now being understood. This is not exaggeration but quite simply what HIV/AIDS has wrought in badly hit African countries in the past twenty years.

Toll in Africa

The epidemic has wreaked havoc in all sectors.

- A large share of Africa's small middle and upper classes have died or have HIV/AIDS, including business-people, civil servants, teachers, miners and military personnel.
- Several African heads of state have lost their children or other relatives, losses that have pushed them to take up prevention in seriousness. The decimation of the most educated and skilled individuals has undermined education, business and even overall development prospects.
- In several countries, one teacher dies every day. In Zambia, where about one in three teachers is infected, fifteen hundred died in 1998 alone.
- In the Central African Republic, more than hundred primary schools closed between 1996 and 1998 because of teachers dying from HIV/AIDS.
- About fifteen per cent of South Africa's bureaucrats are infected.
- Company profits have shrunk because of increases in sick leave, falling productivity, and soaring costs of recruiting and retraining replacements.
- In Zimbabwe, companies are reported to be training seven workers for each job.
- In South Africa, one in five miners is infected with HIV.
- Uganda Railways has lost every tenth employee to HIV/AIDS.
- Workers and businesses in the informal sector are equally badly affected.
- In rural areas too, the deaths of adults has led to shrinking output on both family-run and commercial farms.

Taken together, these numerous costs have eroded the economic development of many African countries. In 1996, HIV/AIDS cost Namibia almost eight per cent of GNP. By 2005, Kenya's GNP is likely to be about fifteen per cent smaller than it would have been without the epidemic. And South Africa's government estimates that HIV/AIDS costs the country two per cent of its GNP each year. By one estimate, over the next twenty years HIV/AIDS will reduce by twenty-five per cent the economies of the African nations south of the Sahara. The epidemic even jeopardises national security. In Uganda, roughly every third person in the military has HIV, and in some other African countries probably every second person. In January 2000, the United Nations Security Council, for the first time moving beyond strict matters of international peace and security, declared that HIV/AIDS was not just a health or humanitarian crisis but a threat to peace in Africa, jeopardising the ability of countries to govern effectively.

And in India ...

Africa's present HIV/AIDS-caused hell is very probably India's future. Crores of young and middle aged Indians infected, sick and dying. Thousands from the wealthy and lakhs from the middle class pushed into poverty. Even larger numbers of the low-income and poor driven into destitution. Countless children orphaned. Villages, communities and even entire generations decimated. Perhaps whole sectors of the economy dislocated and India's development slowed. Our achievements since Independence eroded.

Many signs of this hellish future are already evident in the worst-affected parts of India: fifty lakhs infected; three to five per cent of adults infected in half-a-dozen urban areas; twenty to twenty-five lakhs dead. Just the sickness and death so far has cost India about eleven billion dollars or five per cent of our GNP, in part because the economically vibrant western and southern states have been worst hit. The situation will worsen so rapidly as the lakhs of people already infected get sick and die. The worst-affected states — certainly Maharashtra and Andhra Pradesh, and most likely also Tamil Nadu, Karnataka, Nagaland and Manipur — will in about five to ten years be suffering many aspects of Africa's hellish present. And their problems will continue to snowball because the number of people getting infected will very probably multiply rapidly, particularly in urban areas. Already, the number of Indians infected is doubling every two years or so. And there is no reason to rule out even faster increases. In the African city of Gabarone, for instance, the proportion of all adults infected rose in less than four years from six per cent to nineteen per cent; Pune is already at six per cent, and Namakkal already over that. These worst-hit states will be joined rapidly by other states where the number of people contracting HIV are soaring, such as Delhi, Gujarat, Goa and West Bengal. Not much later, India's remaining states, none of which has done much to prevent HIV/AIDS, will also be badly affected. The first amongst these will probably be Punjab, Himachal Pradesh, Rajasthan, Uttar Pradesh, Bihar and Orissa.

Because HIV/AIDS has already spread deeply in some parts of India it is certain that many of us, or our children or friends or people we know, will contract HIV and so not have a full, long life but will die early and painfully. The dice for these tragedies have already been cast. The number of infected Indians is already so great — particularly in the worst-affected cities and towns in south and west India — that even effective prevention cannot stop many more people from contracting HIV/AIDS. India's epidemic now has a momentum of its own, a juggernaut-like force. Even if the most effective prevention was started today, the number of Indians infected would still increase relentlessly.

There's still time, but not much

But, nonetheless, we still have some power to shape just how bad the epidemic will eventually become. For instance, the World Bank estimates that without successful prevention today the number of Indians infected would eventually (say twenty-five years from now) be nearly twice as large than with effective prevention. So we still have a small and rapidly shrinking window of opportunity — just five to ten years — to prevent the kind of full-blown epidemics that have developed in many African countries. To do this, prevention will have to be done effectively both in the Indian states where levels of infection are already quite high, as well as in every other state to ensure that HIV does not further percolate into people with higher-risk behaviours.

Indians who continue to argue that HIV/AIDS doesn't deserve such importance or so much government money truly miss the point. Of course, some of this confusion arises from the complexities of HIV/AIDS: the lag of six to eight years before infected people get sick, and their death from common diseases. But there is no doubt that HIV/AIDS is factually India's greatest health problem today, as well as a potent threat to our economic and development prospects. Even Prime Minister Vajpayee is convinced of this and has said so publicly. The data and evidence are very clear. And it is equally clear that there is simply no reason why the proportion of Indians infected will not relentlessly climb to the highest levels reached today in Africa: one in three adults, which in India's case would mean over twenty crore people. Anyhow, why assume that money spent on HIV/AIDS prevention is money wasted? The actions and investments required for HIV/AIDS prevention need to be made — should already have been made — irrespective of whether this disease had ever surfaced in India.[2] Our public health system should be drastically improved, especially for the poor. So should our STD services, most so for women. So should our blood supply. Tuberculosis should be made a thing of the past. Sex workers should be emancipated. Illiteracy ended. Poverty and the horrors it breeds done away with. Our laws and policies made more just, especially for disadvantaged or ostracised groups. Our society made more tolerant. All these things should be done anyway, they are part of our constitutional commitment to the welfare of every Indian, they are the milestones by which we should measure our progress. HIV/AIDS just makes it more urgent to achieve these things.

Prevention is the only way to ensure that India's epidemic does not worsen. A vaccine for HIV is still years away, no one knows how long, particularly for the strain of HIV spreading in India. (In the long-term however, the most powerful method for controlling HIV is likely to be an effective vaccine, immunisation which would check the disease in the way that other killer diseases such as smallpox, polio and measles have been controlled and even eradicated.)[3] Medicines

---

2 These actions also need to be taken to prevent hepatitis B, another increasingly important killer STD, which like HIV is transmitted by blood. Though a safe, effective and cheap vaccine exists for hepatitis B, the Indian government has yet to begin mass immunisation with it.

3 The scope for prevention would also be upped by the development of spermicidal or microbicidal products that kill HIV. This would make vaginal or anal sex much safer, as well as allow women greater scope for undertaking prevention without the consent of their male partners. It is expected that such products will be developed in the next few years or so.

to cure AIDS are even more remote. The antiviral drugs currently being used in rich countries are not cures, they delay the onset of disease and death. Anyway, they are too expensive and complex to be used on a wide scale in India, where most people — let alone those impoverished by HIV/AIDS — cannot even afford ordinary medicines.[4] And there are simply no indigenous Indian cures, whether from the ayurveda or unnani systems of medicine. So we cannot hope for a technological breakthrough, a magic bullet. Prevention is the only answer for now. Once India begins to suffer from a widespread epidemic of HIV/AIDS — for instance, ten times the number of people infected today, quite likely in the next five years — the chances of even blunting the epidemic shrink. This is because the destruction caused by the epidemic mounts at a speed that poorer countries like ours simply cannot keep up with. There are the costs of crores of adults and lakhs of infants getting fatally sick. The costs of medicines and of hospital care for them. The costs of lost incomes. The costs of caring for their orphans and other survivors. The costs of attempting prevention with an ever-swelling epidemic. All in all, we must realise that once gripped by a widespread epidemic we will probably not be able to prevent it from continuing to rise to the hellish levels seen in the worst-hit African nations.

It is undeniable that prevention is always extremely difficult. It is difficult to get people to make their sexual behaviours less risky: to always use condoms outside strictly

4 These antiviral drugs stop HIV from replicating and so delay the onset of disease and thus of death. But these drugs must be used in complex multi-drug combinations, require advanced laboratories and monitoring by skilled doctors, and are very expensive. Treatment with these drugs would cost about one lakh rupees per month, affordable only by the very wealthiest Indians.

monogamous relationships, to have STDs treated, and, perhaps, to cut down on the number of partners. It is difficult to achieve such changes in sexual behaviour even with well-educated and affluent people, particularly if there is a culture of silence about sexual matters. It is even more difficult to achieve this with disadvantaged people — whether the poor, women, sex workers or men who have sex with men — because they suffer from multiple vulnerabilities and disadvantages. But it is equally undeniable that prevention can succeed, even in poor developing countries. Perhaps half a dozen low-income or middle-income countries have succeeded in stabilising or slowing the speed at which people are getting infected. These countries are diverse, including Senegal and Uganda in Africa, and Thailand and the Philippines in Asia. There is no reason why India cannot join this list, particularly as we have ample funds for HIV/AIDS prevention.

Our leaders and officials can avoid seriously taking up prevention of HIV/AIDS for as long as they wish but the problem will mount to such a magnitude that address it they must, whether when one crore Indians are infected or dead, or two, five or ten crores. Our problem with HIV/AIDS will not go away, it is here to stay, for ever after it is a factor darkly influencing our and our descendants' sexuality. So address prevention properly, now or later, they must. If they address it now they have some chance of success because the investments of the past fifteen years have created the capacity, at the Centre and in a handful of states, to undertake effective prevention. And these years have also established, from our own experiences and those of other countries, what is needed to make prevention work. If we succeed in realising the following lessons in the next five to ten years, and so achieve prevention of a far-reaching kind, we will very probably have succeeded in preventing a widespread epidemic in India.

What can we do?

Without activism by people like you and me — citizens, the public — the epidemic will flourish. And we need to act now, with foresight, not when it is too late.

- We can have safe sex (and also prevent infection from other routes, such as injecting drugs).
- We can help those close to us learn about sexuality and to practise safe sex.
- We can speak frankly and progressively about sexual matters and so help dispel our society's prejudices and discomfort about sexuality; in short, make this once again the land of the *Kama Sutra*.
- We can support or work with the fine organisations working to prevent HIV/AIDS, caring for the sick, bringing together people with HIV/AIDS, or protecting the rights of those infected or from disadvantaged groups.
- We can protest with vigour against abuse of the rights of people with HIV/AIDS or of disadvantaged groups.
- We can be truly compassionate towards those with HIV/AIDS and join them in their fight for survival and dignity.
- We can expect our politicians and bureaucrats — and every other kind of leader, whether the heads of media organisations, the heads of religions or our favourite film stars — to champion HIV/AIDS prevention in the most progressive way.
- We can push our state and central government to do what truly needs to be done to protect every Indian, however poor or reviled by our society, from contracting HIV.

- We can make HIV/AIDS prevention into a political issue by which we judge the performance of political parties, particularly at the state level. We can make our leaders and government realise that they are accountable for their inaction, for every infection and death that takes place while they are in power.

What governments must do

Political leadership is an essential prerequisite to true HIV/AIDS prevention. This is obvious from the experience of the few developing countries that have succeeded in prevention. It is also apparent from the relative success of Tamil Nadu — where prevention has been led by the chief minister and senior bureaucrats — and the failures of virtually every other Indian state, including badly affected ones like Maharashtra, Andhra Pradesh and, increasingly, Delhi. If our prime minister, president, chief ministers, other senior ministers and members of Parliament do not come forward and become advocates of HIV/AIDS prevention, our efforts are doomed, irrespective of how much money they spend on HIV/AIDS. These leaders will need to do much more than pay lip-service to this cause.

- They will need to talk frankly and sympathetically about sex and sexuality, about STDs and HIV, about sex workers, men who have sex with men, drug injectors.

- They will have to physically embrace people with HIV/AIDS, to eat and drink with them, so that everyone understands that this disease is not spread by ordinary contact, that there are no reasons to fear or discriminate against those infected or sick. Could any message be more powerful than this: "If the prime minister or chief minister can do it, embrace and eat with a sex worker with AIDS, so can I!"

- They will need to encourage men and women to use condoms, to get their STDs treated, to learn about safe sexual behaviours.
- They will need to fight for explicit and powerful awareness campaigns, in the mass media, in schools, in colleges.
- They will have to champion the rights of women, of sex workers, of men who have sex with men, of prisoners, and most, of people with HIV/AIDS. They will have to fight for the legal and policy changes needed to achieve this.
- They will have to ensure that the persecution or abuse of people with HIV/AIDS or of those with higher-risk behaviours is ended.
- They will have to persuade religious, business, media, entertainment and other leaders to take up prevention as a cause.

In short, they will have to make HIV/AIDS prevention into a cause that has political and public commitment.

Terror does not work

But prevention will fail if HIV/AIDS remains a cause of stigma, of discrimination, of terror. Prevention of HIV/AIDS is very difficult at the best of times; but it is an impossibility in a climate of discrimination and terror. The irrational dread of this disease — which turns into cruelty and discrimination against those infected, sick, or accused of being at "higher-risk" — is the greatest impediment to prevention. Removing this dread, and thus removing the discrimination that results, is a precondition to effective prevention. This lesson is bitterly evident from Maharashtra's failure to prevent a widespread epidemic of HIV/AIDS. This state's prevention efforts have been undermined by the terror and fear that result from the coercive policies still advocated by its politicians, judges, police and even some health officials. If Maharashtra and other states decide to erase the stigma and terror currently attached to HIV/AIDS, they will have to do many things to rectify the situation. (The stigma and terror do not vanish on their own; they are cripplingly strong even in the worst-hit African countries.)

- Their political leaders will have to understand why coercion does not work, and to forswear this approach.
- Awareness campaigns will have to portray HIV/AIDS as just a disease, not death.
- Those who seek voluntary counselling and testing will have to be ensured complete confidentiality or anonymity.
- People from "higher-risk groups" and those with HIV/AIDS will have to be reassured that coercion and discrimination have truly ended.
- And people with HIV/AIDS will have to be treated as responsible citizens, not as criminals whose rights are limited by do's and don'ts about marriage, child-bearing and other issues.

Early prevention

Prevention needs to be taken up early. Andhra Pradesh is a good lesson of what happens if effective prevention is not started early. In the past half-decade it has gone from having very few cases of HIV to having, with Maharashtra, the largest proportion of its people infected with HIV. Karnataka is doing no better. The lesson for those fortunate Indian states that have very few infected people now, or where infections are still concentrated in those with higher-risk behaviours, is very clear: start prevention right away. It is only a matter of time before HIV spreads widely and then multiplies in the larger public.

Eight steps

There are interventions specific to HIV/AIDS prevention that need to be put in place. These need to be made available to the larger public and, in an even more concentrated way, to every "higher-risk" and vulnerable group, certainly including men who have sex with men. These are:

- Condom promotion and distribution.
- Treatment of STDs.
- Access to clean syringes and needles for injecting drug users.
- HIV/AIDS and sexual health education campaigns for the public and, especially, all teenagers.
- Face-to-face education for those at higher risk.
- Voluntary counselling and anonymous testing services.
- In the medical field, there needs to be rigorous screening of blood and blood products, and strict implementation of universal precautions in medical settings.
- The guarantee that health staff will not discriminate against those with HIV/AIDS.

Sex education

The public education campaigns on HIV/AIDS need to reach young people, anybody from age ten or so up. They are the next generation of sexually active people and so at greatest risk of HIV. Already, in several parts of India where the epidemic has moved from its first phase in "higher-risk groups" into the "lower-risk" population, a sizeable and ever-increasing share of infections are in young people. To be effective these campaigns need to be frank because India's young suffer from a crippling lack of parental advice and scientific information on sex.

Those worried that sex education will promote sexual activity should rest their fears. Research from across the world shows that sex education has no effect on the amount of sexual activity or the age that youngsters begin sex; it leads only to safer sex.

Anyhow, which of us would not prefer that our children learn about these sensitive issues from trained and responsible people rather than from tragedy? It is imperative that sex education be started as early as possible. Teachers at schools and colleges should be trained to teach sex education to create a better understanding of STD, HIV/AIDS, condom use, abortions, homosexuality, and of how to negotiate safe sex. And innovative approaches must be used to reach the many Indian children or adolescents who do not go to school or college, or are illiterate. In all these efforts, good values can be inculcated, but it is essential that the stress on morals not prevent teaching the basic facts. Young people are going to take risks anyway — whether smoking or sex — so it is best to promote safer behaviours by providing them the information in as non-judgemental a way as possible.

Indians more likely to get HIV

The vulnerabilities that affect the overwhelming majority of Indians need to be reduced because the average Indian, whether male or female, middle class or poor, is vulnerable to HIV/AIDS in too many ways.

- Our society-wide discomfort about sex, sexuality, sexual health; anything to do with sex.
- Our refusal to accept that many men frequent sex workers or have sex with other men.
- The lack of information for young people about sexuality, safe sex and STD prevention.
- Poverty.
- The terrible situation of women.
- Illiteracy.
- The lack of even basic health care, including treatment for STDs and tuberculosis.
- The laws and public attitudes that lead to the oppression of vilified groups, whether sex workers, men who have sex with men or drug users.

HIV/AIDS will continue to thrive if these vulnerabilities are not greatly reduced. Unfortunately, too many policy makers think that HIV can be stopped simply by providing specific interventions, such as condoms or education, without tackling vulnerabilities. They argue for this limited agenda on the flimsiest of evidence. If anything, the evidence points in the opposite direction, to the need for addressing vulnerabilities as well as providing access to HIV/AIDS or STD-specific programmes. The conclusive proof that vulnerabilities have to be addressed comes from the fact that industrialised countries have successfully avoided HIV/AIDS epidemics while developing countries, all of which suffer from myriad vulnerabilities, have largely failed.

Sonagachi shows the way

The lesson about the need to reduce vulnerabilities applies even more to "higher-risk groups": only those efforts work that address the causes of their vulnerability. "Higher-risk groups" need effective prevention most urgently because they are at great risk themselves of getting infected and of transmitting HIV to others. Consider sex workers. In India and elsewhere, they have been and remain amongst the greatest victims of HIV/AIDS and of the terrible coercion in the name of prevention. Programmes for sex workers in Maharashtra, Gujarat, Delhi and most other states — and to a lesser degree even in Tamil Nadu — have failed miserably because almost nothing has been done to reduce the oppression of these women at the hands of brothel-keepers, pimps, mafia and police. But in Calcutta's Sonagachi "red light" area, HIV and STD levels have been kept low because sex workers have been allowed to unionise and so to battle the causes of their vulnerability. Once unionised, they have demanded and secured improvements in health care and STD treatment services, collectively forced customers to use condoms, tackled police harassment, and started education programmes for their children and savings schemes for themselves. Moreover, in the Netherlands and other areas where sex work is legitimate and sex workers have civil and workers' rights, they have impressively low HIV rates. While it is obvious that there cannot be a single simple answer to solving the web of poverty, violence, mob exploitation, police and political connivance, trafficking and sexual slavery that characterises India's sex work scene, there is every reason to shape prevention around what sex workers themselves think will work. Anyhow, the very clear lesson is that you cannot have unchanged persecution and poverty and yet expect sex workers — or men who have sex with men or injecting drug users or street children — to adopt safe behaviours and so to stop themselves and others from contracting HIV. Unfortunately, barring Sonagachi and a few other limited projects, almost nothing has been done in India to reduce the vulnerabilities faced by particularly disadvantaged groups.

The final lesson concerns the relationship between Indian men and women. It is a relationship marked by such terrible inequality that marriage is the act that puts many women at risk of HIV. Indian men need to be more responsible vis-à-vis women; for this, a change in public values has to be encouraged. (This is not to blame Indian men for the epidemic — even more men than women are infected and dying themselves.) But even more urgent, Indian women need legal and policy support to have greater economic and social independence. At least part of the reason why industrialised countries have prevented epidemics of HIV/AIDS is because women possess significant social and economic independence from men, which allows them to negotiate safe sex.

It is only if we achieve prevention of this far-reaching kind that we will spare ourselves and countless other Indians from the horrors of HIV/AIDS. The barriers to our succeeding are enormous. The odds are stacked against us because our government, and we as a society, have done badly on too many development issues in the past fifty years, whether poverty, literacy, health or the situation of women. And we have failed on HIV/AIDS for the past fifteen years. But we have to succeed and that too succeed now, because the alternative — failure — is a horrific prospect. If we fail we suffer what much of Africa is suffering today.

For the next decade or until we know prevention is truly working, you and I will everyday be dogged by some bitter uncertainties. Will Africa's tragedy with HIV/AIDS be India's future? Will India eventually be equally savagely decimated by HIV/AIDS? Will your life or my life — or of how many of our relatives, children, family, friends — have been ravaged by this disease? Will the lives of crores of other Indians have been ravaged?

ANNEXE

A Kama Sutra for the Age of AIDS: How to have Safer Sex

While abstaining completely from sex with others is obviously the surest way of ensuring that one does not contract HIV from the sexual route, this is not an attractive option for most people. A more feasible and very effective option is to have an absolutely monogamous relationship with an uninfected partner.

But for those of us for whom neither of these options work, with some basic precautions sex can be as much fun in the age of AIDS as at the time the *Kama Sutra* was penned. In fact, if you consistently maintain these basic precautions, there is simply no reason why you cannot be an expert in the entire *Kama Sutra*. So read on carefully.

The overwhelming majority of HIV infections, about eighty to ninety per cent of the global total, occur from unprotected vaginal or anal intercourse with an infected partner, whether it is sex between men and women or between men and other men. (Sex between women — lesbian sex — only rarely leads to HIV transmission.) Transmission of HIV takes place during sex because HIV is found in sperm, vaginal fluids and blood (including menstrual fluids), and the virus can enter the body through the lining of the vagina, vulva, penis or rectum during sex. A single act of unprotected sexual intercourse with an infected partner is sufficient to contract HIV. "Unprotected" intercourse means intercourse without a latex condom, typically a condom for men.[1]

As people infected with HIV do not develop symptoms of illness for years, there is no way of knowing whether one's sexual partner is infected unless he or she has never engaged in any risky behaviour or has been repeatedly tested for the virus. Hence, unless you are having a monogamous relationship with a person whom you know is not infected, you must assume that every person is infected and you must have safer sex with them.[2] Remember! There is simply no way to tell

1 Latex is a material made from rubber. Up till recently, the male condom was the only method available for protection against STDs. The female condom is a recent alternative. It is a plastic sheath that a woman unfolds and inserts into her vagina. Just like a male condom, it is effective both as a contraceptive and protection against STDs. Unfortunately, female condoms are barely available anywhere in India, not even in many major cities. Scientists are also trying to develop liquids or gels that can kill HIV if placed in the vagina or anus, but none are likely to be widely available for several more years.

2 Even two HIV-infected people should have safe sex with one another. This is essential to preventing "re-infection" with HIV, where an already infected person contracts a more damaging or treatment-resistant form of the virus. And it is also essential to prevent infection with other STDs, which people with HIV/AIDS are more vulnerable to because of their weakened immune systems.

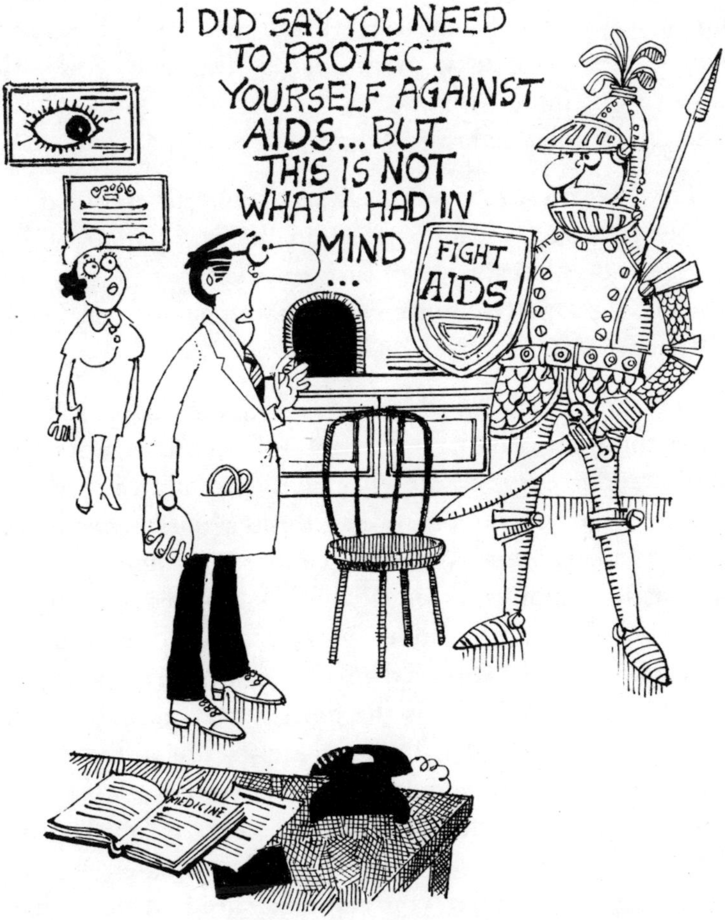
I DID SAY YOU NEED TO PROTECT YOURSELF AGAINST AIDS... BUT THIS IS NOT WHAT I HAD IN MIND ...
FIGHT AIDS
MEDICINE

from a person's physical appearance whether he or she is infected with HIV. And only trained doctors can tell whether a person has AIDS, and even this requires clinical examination and typically a confirmatory HIV test. So don't assume that because a person is sexy, good-looking, healthy or young that they are not infected.

Here is what safer sex means.

- First, whenever having vaginal or anal intercourse, you or your partner must use a good quality male latex condom. A new condom must be used each time you have intercourse. When used properly, condoms are very effective in preventing HIV transmission.

- You may or may not wish to add extra water-based lubricant to the condom while having vaginal intercourse. But during anal intercourse it is absolutely essential to lubricate both the anus itself and the condom, even if this is a lubricated condom, as most Indian brands are now. Unlike the vagina, the anus lacks natural lubricants or expanding muscles and there is great risk that the condom will tear without additional lubrication. Only water-based lubricants or contraceptive jellies should be used. KY Jelly is the most widely available water-based lubricant in India. Unfortunately, even in the metros, contraceptive or spermicidal jellies are scarce, even in large pharmacies. Never put oil, vaseline, butter or ghee as a lubricant; these oil-based lubricants only increase the risk of the condom tearing. If you can't get hold of water-based lubricants or a contraceptive jelly, use saliva or water; they don't damage condoms, though of course they don't provide much lubrication. To further reduce the risks during anal sex, some men use two condoms, one on top of another, with water-based lubricant added to both condoms.

🎗 Oral sex on a man's penis poses some but low risks of HIV transmission to the person who is sucking. There is no risk at all to the person whose penis is being sucked. The risk increases if sperm is taken into one's mouth or swallowed; so don't allow this. If you want to be entirely safe during oral sex with a man it is advisable to use a condom. Another effective prevention method is to not put the tip of the penis within one's mouth, but to only lick and suck the glans, the shaft and the testicles, strictly avoiding the "pee-hole." Avoid oral sex without a condom if you have cuts or tears in your mouth, have a sore throat, have just brushed or flossed, or been to the dentist.

🎗 The risks of contracting HIV from oral sex on a woman's vagina are lower than oral sex on a man, particularly if this is not practised during menstruation. To be completely safe, cut open a condom and use this as a barrier between your mouth and the vagina.

🎗 Oral-anal contact — putting one's mouth or tongue to the anus — poses no risks of HIV transmission. But it does effectively spread other serious diseases, such as hepatitis B, amoebas and parasites. Again, use a cut condom as a barrier between your mouth and the anus.

🎗 Kissing on the mouth has such low risk that it is considered almost entirely safe: this is because HIV is only barely present in saliva and is also killed by elements in it and in the stomach. There is risk if either partner's mouth is bleeding or has cuts or sores. There is possibly some slight risk with prolonged "French" or deep kissing, where people tongue each other's mouths. But licking or kissing a person's face or body anywhere — apart from the penis head or vagina — is completely safe.

So is masturbating or caressing oneself or others: there is no risk at all of contracting or passing HIV.

🎗 If you use sex toys like vibrators or dildoes, don't share them as this can spread HIV. If you are going to share them, put a condom on them, or clean them properly with soap and hot water after each use.

🎗 Finally, beyond condoms and avoiding the riskiest forms of oral sex, safer sex involves having STDs treated. This is so because the risk of transmitting or contracting HIV is especially high if either you or your partner suffer from other STDs, as these typically multiply the efficiency of HIV transmission. Most STDs are curable with common antibiotics, and such treatment enormously reduces the risks of HIV transmission.[3] The most common signs of STD infection include discharge from the penis in men; abnormal discharge from the vagina in women; blisters, sores or lumps around the genitals or anus; swollen glands in the groin; and increased frequency in urinating or pain in doing so. So if you are suffering from any of these symptoms, don't be embarrassed and seek medical care promptly; it may save you or your partner from contracting HIV. In fact, sexually active people should consult a doctor about any suspicious rash or sore in the genital area. Remember that most STDs are easily transmitted by oral sex, and that condoms are not always

3 However, because many STDs cause none or only mild symptoms, especially in women, many people don't even realise that they are infected. When untreated, STDs may cause serious complications, such as chronic abdominal pain, infertility and stillbirth in women. Syphilis, for instance, may be passed on to a developing baby in the womb, and cause premature birth, blindness and even the death of the baby.

effective in preventing transmission of some STDs, particularly genital herpes and warts.

🎗 One last word of advice. Apart from ignorance, the major reasons why people don't consistently have safer sex are because they aren't prepared and because they feel awkward about negotiating this. The solution is to prepare and to practise. Whether you are a man or woman, heterosexual or homosexual, prepare by keeping condoms handy if you are expecting to have sex. And if you are expecting to have anal sex, remember to keep lubricants or contraceptive jellies handy too. Get over your embarrassment about buying these things by going to shops outside your neighbourhood. Make sure the condom is not old — preferably no older than two years since manufacture — damaged or brittle. Learn to carry condoms and lubricants with you when you travel or when you go to parties or to other places where you might end up having sex. Keep the condoms protected from heat, sharp objects and finger-nails. Never test the condom by inflating or stretching it.

🎗 And practise! Practise asking, in a relaxed unthreatening way, your partner to use a condom; or telling them that you wish to use one. Practise being firm and insistent about this, irrespective of whatever they say or wish. Practise saying "No!" to unsafe sex. Practise putting on a condom correctly on yourself or your partner. Practise doing this in the dark or in whatever setting you might have sex. Practise smearing lubricant on the condom or on the anus or vagina. Practise taking off the condom from yourself or your partner. Practise how you or your partner can make oral sex safer. And practise discussing sexual issues, particularly HIV/AIDS and other STDs, with your partner in a way that doesn't destroy the romance or eroticism.

Put the condom on an erect penis before beginning intercourse. When you put a condom on, hold the small nipple at the end of the condom and unroll the condom on the penis. Keep the nipple gently pinched so that when the person wearing the condom ejaculates, there is space for the ejaculated sperm, and it doesn't split the condom. If you're really worried about breakage, you can also pull out of your partner before ejaculation, even with a condom on. After ejaculation, make sure that the condom does not come off the penis; hold the condom firmly against the penis during withdrawal. After tying a knot in the used condom, dispose it of in a plastic or paper bag.

Understanding HIV/AIDS

Apart from the sexual route, there are only two other routes for HIV to spread: by contaminated blood, and from an infected mother to her foetus or infant.

There are absolutely no other means for the spread of HIV. Saliva, sweat, tears, urine or faeces do not spread HIV. So HIV cannot be spread through casual contact, whether this involves the sharing of food or drinking utensils, towels or bedding, toilets, or swimming in a pool. And HIV cannot pass through intact external skin, through the air or water, or be carried by mosquitoes or other biting insects. In this sense, HIV is not a "contagious" disease like the flu, tuberculosis, polio, measles, cholera or diarrhoea — which are spread through the air, water or contaminated eatables — or malaria or dengue fever, which are spread through mosquitoes.

Exposure to HIV-infected blood, blood products or organs transmits HIV. Transmission through the blood route takes place in a number of ways. One major way is through transfusion of blood, blood products or human organs contaminated with HIV.

- Another important cause is the sharing of syringes or needles by intravenous drug users.

- And another is the reuse in medical settings — such as hospitals or immunisation campaigns — of contaminated medical, surgical or dental equipment, ranging from syringes and needles to surgical knives. Though this is not an important source of infection in industrialised countries, it is a significant problem in India and many other developing countries because medical equipment is very often not properly sterilised. Finally, HIV is transmitted by common skin-piercing instruments, for instance, those used in piercing the nose or ears, tattooing or even blades used by barbers on more than one person. Overall, in India and many other poor countries, transmission through the blood-borne route is responsible for about eight to ten per cent of HIV infections.

- The third and last transmission route is from an infected mother to her foetus or infant during pregnancy, birth or breastfeeding. An HIV-infected mother in a developing country faces a twenty-five to forty-five per cent risk of passing the infection to her baby during pregnancy or labour. Breastfeeding by an infected mother adds a risk of fifteen per cent or more, depending on how long breastfeeding is carried on for and other factors that scientists are trying to understand. So, on an average, in countries like India where almost all mothers breastfeed, every third or even second child born to HIV-infected mothers is likely to be infected. Treatment of infected mothers-to-be and their new-born infants with the drugs zidovudine (AZT) or nevirapine can dramatically reduce the risks of the child being infected before or during birth, and to some degree also against infection from breastfeeding. Treatment with AZT currently costs about Rs 10,000. In the many African countries with large proportions of their population infected with HIV, mother-to-child transmission is responsible for about ten per cent of infections. Infected children get sick and die much sooner than adults because their immune system is far weaker; in developing countries children usually die by the age of five.

🎗 Until today, typical medical solutions to epidemics — a vaccine to prevent infection or medicines to treat or cure the disease — have not yet been discovered for HIV/AIDS. Since there is no vaccine for HIV, the only way to prevent infection is to avoid behaviours that put a person at risk of infection, such as having unprotected sex.

🎗 HIV acts slowly in adults. For around six to eight years after the initial infection, most adults remain healthy and usually have no symptoms.[4] During this stage, HIV can only be detected by HIV-specific blood, saliva or urine tests.[5]

---

4 Most people can expect to survive for eight to ten years from the initial infection. But the course of disease can vary greatly. A few people die within two years of being infected. About four to seven per cent survive beyond twenty years.

5 Most of the tests now used in private or government testing centres are reliable, with the blood tests being the most reliable. Typically, a second test is done to confirm a first positive result. Testing should only be done at reliable centres, with trained laboratory staff. It is important to remember that for a "window period" of three to twelve weeks following infection, tests will fail to pick up antibodies to HIV, which is what the tests measure.

People who are "positive" to these tests but are still to develop symptoms are typically called HIV-positive or asymptomatic.

It is very important to realise that contracting HIV is not the end of life, it is not an immediate death sentence. From the time of infection, most people can expect to live six to eight years healthily and normally, especially if they have decent nutrition and preventive health care. In these years they can even undertake strenuous activity. In the US, for instance, star basketball player Magic Johnson continued to play in competitions for several years after being diagnosed with HIV. And even after developing AIDS, with good treatment for the diseases that occur, one can be assured of several more years of life.

From the initial infection onwards, HIV continues to actively multiply, infecting and killing cells of the immune system. Over the years, as the immune system deteriorates, a variety of complications begin to surface. These are often experienced months to years before the life-threatening diseases that make up the syndrome known as AIDS. These symptoms include large lymph nodes or "swollen glands" that may be enlarged for months, lack of energy, weight loss, frequent fevers and sweats, persistent oral or vaginal fungal infections, skin rashes, pelvic inflammatory disease that does not respond to treatment, or short-term memory loss. Some people develop severe herpes infections that cause mouth, genital or anal sores, or a painful nerve disease known as shingles. Children may have delayed development or simply not thrive. Sometimes, people are so weakened by these symptoms that they do not have the energy to do household chores or to go to work.

🎗 In developing countries it typically takes six to eight years after the initial infection for HIV to multiply to the point where it makes the body's immune system too weak to fend off diseases.[6] This advanced stage of immune deficiency is known as AIDS.[7]

🎗 People with AIDS develop a variety of increasingly more frequent and ferocious illnesses. These eventually prove fatal. Because AIDS is a syndrome, the illnesses vary a great deal, depending on the individual and on the illnesses common in that area or country. People with AIDS often suffer from multiple illness at a time. In India, tuberculosis, pneumonia, chronic diarrhoea, severe weight loss, ferocious eye and skin infections, chronic herpes and oral fungal infections are the most common AIDS-related illnesses. An increasing number of Indians with AIDS are contracting kala azar, especially in Bihar and UP. But rare types of cancers, pneumonia and diseases of the brain and central nervous system also occur. These are rarely identified in India because of the poor state of medical diagnostic services. The illnesses that people with AIDS suffer from are known as opportunistic infections, as they take advantage of the damaged immune system. Many of these diseases rarely affect healthy people. In people with

6 Preventive treatment for tuberculosis and several other HIV-related diseases will help postpone the development of sickness in HIV-infected people.

7 Though the term AIDS is popularly used, for medical purposes it has been replaced by stage-by-stage classifications of HIV infection. AIDS refers only to the very late stages of immune suppression. In poor countries, most people die of opportunistic infections caused by advanced HIV infection even before they develop AIDS. In other words, they die of "HIV disease." But this distinction is not important to us, only to researchers and doctors.

AIDS, however, these infections are severe and often fatal because the immune system is so weakened.

- Because many of the symptoms of AIDS-related illnesses are not specific to AIDS — for instance, TB or diarrhoea — doctors confirm that a patient has AIDS either when several major indications of AIDS are evident, or by testing for the presence of HIV. And because people with AIDS typically die from common diseases, their deaths are rarely recognised or recorded as being caused by AIDS.

- Treatment of AIDS consists of treating these illnesses with antibiotics. With prompt diagnosis and good nutrition, people with AIDS will recover from some bouts of illnesses. Hence, people with AIDS may experience bouts of life-threatening illness followed by disease-free periods. Eventually, of course, the immune system is too far damaged and the person succumbs to some illness. In India and other countries with bad health systems, many people die within six months to one year of first developing severe illnesses. But those who can ensure good treatment, care and nutrition, may survive for several years. And a handful of very wealthy Indians can afford the very expensive multi-drug or "cocktail" therapies that delay the development of AIDS and so allow HIV-positive people to live much longer and healthier lives than they would otherwise.[8]

- There are simply no cures for HIV/AIDS in the Indian systems of medicines such as unnani or ayurveda, and people should not waste their money on alleged cures.

8 Treatment with these medications costs about Rs 1 lakh per month and requires very good monitoring and supervision by skilled doctors. The most effective treatments are combination therapies of three antiviral drugs. Monotherapy with a single antiviral is not recommended.

It is very important to remember that even when a person has AIDS, he or she poses NO risks to others and there is no reason at all to avoid, discriminate against or quarantine them. HIV itself cannot be spread by normal contact. Nor can healthy people contract the diseases that people with AIDS suffer from. TB is the only important exception, requiring obvious precautions such as a complete course of treatment, not going to work or school, sleeping in a separate room, and avoiding close contact with others, especially children. After two or three weeks of sustained treatment, people with TB are no longer infectious to others, though a doctor should judge this.

BIBLIOGRAPHY

There is now a huge amount of academic and policy writing on HIV/AIDS in India. The most important materials referred to in this book are listed here, particularly those that would be useful to readers of this book.

AIDS

"Prostitution and HIV." Neil McKeganey. 1994, 8: 1215-1226.

"HIV and men who have sex with men: perspectives from selected Asian countries." Chan, Kavi et al. 1998, 12, 559-568.

"HIV/AIDS in India: a country responds to a challenge." Salunke SR, Shaukat M, Hira SK, Jagtap MR. 1998, 12S; S27-S31.3

AIDS Analysis Asia

"Special survey of Tamil Nadu." January 1995.

AIDS Bhedbhav Virodhi Andolan
(*AIDS Anti-Discrimination Movement*)

Women and AIDS, 1990.

AIDS and Manav Adhikaron Ka Sankat, 1991.

The Blood of the Professionals, 1991.

Less than Gay, 1991.

Hard Times for Positive Travel, 1993.

Needle of Suspicion, 1996. (*Thought-provoking reports from an independent NGO.*)

AIDS Weekly Plus
"Industry in India to fight AIDS through workplace." Keith Key. April 1 1996, 17.
"Expanding AIDS epidemic in India includes monógamous wives." Sandra W Key, DeNoon et al. May 1 1998, 10.
"Compulsory testing sends HIV/AIDS underground." Sandra W Key, DeNoon et al. September 3 1998, 15.
Asiaweek
"Children for Sale." Ruchira Gupta. March 1 1996.
Bloom, David; Godwin, Peter; (editors)
The Economics of HIV and AIDS: the case of South and South East Asia. Oxford University Press. 1997. (*Thorough.*)
British Overseas Development Administration
Review of Best Practice for Interventions in Sexual Health. Edited by Peter Gordon and Carolyn Sleightholme. (*Very useful for planners.*)
Dube, Siddharth
"AIDS: It's Here." *Sunday*. August 25 1991.
"Facade of AIDS Prevention?" *Economic and Political Weekly*. April 11 1992.
"The rising cost of AIDS." Choices. UN Development Programme, 1993.
The Prescriber: Special issue on HIV/AIDS prevention, treatment and care. (Editor) UNICEF, September 1998.
Economic and Political Weekly
"HIV/AIDS in India: gulf between rhetoric and reality." Radhika Ramasubban. November 7 1998. (*Excellent analysis.*)
Economic Times
"Special report: I. An Ailing System. II. Prisoners of the Death Cell." Shailendra. January 28 1996.
Financial Express
"Chemists body to take up AIDS drug's selective distribution with Cipla, Glaxo." Anju Ghangurde. June 7 1999.
Financial Times
"The slow poisoner: India refuses to panic over its growing AIDS epidemic." Krishna Guha. October 9 1999.

Godwin, Peter (editor)
The Looming Epidemic: the impact of HIV and AIDS in India. Mosaic Books. 1998. (*Very useful.*)

Harvard AIDS Review
AIDS in India, Fall 1995. (*See especially the excellent series by Jaya Sreedhar.*)

Health Policy
"Impact of HIV/AIDS on the national economy of India." K. Anand et al. 1999, 47, 195-205.

Hira, Subhash et al.
"Clinical spectrum of HIV/AIDS in the Asia-Pacific region." AIDS. 1998, 12, 145-154.
"Evidence of AIDS-related mortality in Mumbai, India." The Lancet. October 3 1999, Vol 354, 1175.

Hubley, John; Chowdhury, Shankar; Chandramouli, V.
AIDS Handbook: A guide to the understanding of AIDS and HIV. Popular Prakashan. 1995. (*Sensible and detailed advice that will be tremendously useful to parents, teachers, counsellors and grassroot workers in India.*)

Indian Express
"Students' hangout — Red-light areas." Anuradha Nagaraj. December 2 1992.

India Today
"The Indian face of AIDS." Harinder Baweja and Arun Katiyar. November 30 1991.
"Putting life on the line." Vijay Jung Thapa and Lekha Rattanani. August 31 1995.
"AIDS: Striking Home." Farah Baria. March 15 1997.
"Sex workers: legal soliciting." Udayan Namboodiri and Nandita Chowdhury. December 8 1997.
"Emphatic Campaign: fight for justice by sex workers." M.G. Radhakrishnan. March 15 1999.
"Prayer and Precaution." Stephen David. May 10 1999.

InterPress News Service (IPS)
"AIDS: Street Children Are Most Vulnerable." Bijoy Basant Patro. September 3 1997.

"Legal Luminaries Seek AIDS Legislation." Mitu Varma. October 21 1997.

"Election Fever Bypasses 'HIV Village'." R. Dev Raj. March 1 1998.

"HIV/AIDS Prompts Scramble for Aid." R. Dev Raj. May 27 1998.

"HIV Compels Sex Education in Indian Schools." R. Dev Raj. November 19 1998.

Khan, Shivananda (editor)

South Asia regional consultation meeting on male reproductive and sexual health and HIV/AIDS for males who have sex with males. Naz Foundation International. March 1999.

Labour File

Fatal ignorance: HIV/AIDS in Workplace. (*An outstanding collection of articles on the impact of HIV/AIDS on poorer workers in the informal industrial sector.*)

Lancet

"HIV Epidemic in India." Jain M, John TJ. 1996; 348:412-413.2.

Lawyers Collective

Various issues of this excellent newsletter focused on the legal aspects of HIV/AIDS.

Los Angeles Times

"Superstition, Poverty May Bring AIDS Crisis in India." Mark Fineman. May 28 1990.

McDermott, Jim

Report to the Speaker of the US House of Representatives: the AIDS Epidemic in Asia. June 6 1991.

National AIDS Control Organisation.

India Country Scenario 1997-98.

Current Status and Trends of HIV/AIDS Epidemic in India, October 1999.

High Risk Behaviour Study from 18 Cities. Mala Sinha, compiler. (No date given.)

Nag, Moni

Sexual Behaviour and Aids in India. Vikas. 1996.

The Nation

"India's Shame: Sexual Slavery and Political Corruption." Robert Friedman. April 8 1996.

National Public Radio
AIDS in Asia Series on "All Things Considered." Transcript. 17 Feb-6 March 1994.
Newsweek International
"India: Red-Light Revolution." Sudip Mazumdar. February 15 1999.
Social Science and Medicine
"Health-seeking strategies and sexual health among female sex workers in urban India." Catrin Evans and Helen Lambert. Volume 44, No 12, 1791-1803.
The AIDS Reader
"AIDS Care in India." Sarman Singh. 1997, 7(3):101-106.
UNAIDS
Country Profile India: HIV/AIDS, December 1998.
AIDS Epidemic update: December 1999.
Vajpayee, Atal Bihari
Address by the Prime Minister at the National Programme for Prevention and Control of HIV/AIDS, December 12 1998.
World Bank
Staff Appraisal Report India National AIDS Control Project. March 9 1992.
Project Appraisal Document for the Second National HIV/AIDS Control Project, May 13 1999.
Confronting AIDS: Public priorities in a global epidemic. 1997.

International

Aggleton, Peter (editor)
Bisexualities and AIDS: international perspectives. Taylor & Francis. 1996, 234.
Beyrer, Chris
War in the Blood: Sex, Politics and AIDS in South-East Asia. Zed Books. 1998. (*Outstanding analysis of the dynamics in Southeast Asia.*)
Boston Globe
"AIDS and the African: A Continent's Crisis." October 10-13 1999. (*A four-part series.*)

Chicago Tribune

"Africa — the ailing continent." Paul Salopek. January 2000. (*Excellent three-part series.*)

The Economist

"Poor man's plague." September 21 1991.

"An ounce of prevention." July 4 1998.

"Orphans of the virus." August 14 1999.

Foreman, Martin (editor)

AIDS and Men: Taking risks or taking responsibility? Zed Books. 1999. (*Excellent discussion of this important issue.*)

Garrett, Laurie

The Coming Plague: Newly emerging diseases in a world out of balance. Penguin, 1995.

Mann, Jonathan; Tarantola, Daniel et al (editors)

AIDS in the World I: A Global Report Harvard University Press. 1992.

AIDS in the World II: A Global Report. Edited by Mann and Tarantola. Oxford University Press. 1996.

(*Encyclopedic and thorough, excellent as reference sources.*)

New York Times

"AIDS in Africa: A killer rages on." Erik Eckholm. Four part series beginning September 16 1990.

"In Africa, a Deadly Silence About AIDS Is Lifting." Lawrence Altman. July 13 1999.

Schoofs, Mark

"AIDS: the agony of Africa." The Village Voice. November-December 1999. (*This prize-winning eight-part series is perhaps the best journalism on the subject. Available on the Web at www.villagevoice.com*)

Shilts, Randy

And the Band Played On: politics, people and the AIDS epidemic. Viking Penguin. 1988.

Washington Post

"Facing a Global AIDS Crisis." Princeton N. Lyman. August 11 1999.

"AIDS is security threat Gore tells UN Council." Colum Lynch. January 10 2000.

FOR MORE INFORMATION AND HELP

This is a rough guide to organisations in India working on HIV/AIDS, as well as to international sources that are accessible and reliable. It is not comprehensive, nor do I necessarily mean to recommend any organisation.

The National AIDS Control Organisation is at the Ministry of Health, Nirman Bhawan, New Delhi-110 001. Ph 3017706. Fax 3793320. Email www.nic.in/naco.

NACO has set up AIDS Helplines in major cities. Dialling **1097** in Calcutta, Chandigarh, Delhi and several other cities will get you anonymous information and counselling on HIV/AIDS. This service is available round the clock and is free of charge. Callers calling from a public telephone booth do not need to pay money. Information is provided through a voice response system linked to the computer. People who ask for individual counselling are referred to non-governmental organisations or hospitals.

The most comprehensive source of information on all aspects of HIV/AIDS is UNAIDS, the Joint United Nations Programme on HIV/AIDS. They produce an enormous range of technical, policy, advocacy and information material. These are available from the UNAIDS office in Delhi, which also maintains an information centre of other materials. Contact them at 55 Lodi Estate, New Delhi 110003. Ph 4649892 or 4628877. Fax 4649895. Email unaids.in@undp.org. The UNAIDS website is at www.unaids.org. There is also an India-specific website at www.unaids.org.in

Other Internet and email sources

For an excellent email service focused on HIV/AIDS in South and SE Asia, subscribe to Sea-aids by sending them an email at healthdev@hivnet.ch or go to www.unaidsapict.inet.co.th or www.hivnet.ch

The US Centers for Disease Control are an extremely reliable source of information and data on many aspects of HIV/AIDS. www.cdc.gov/nchstp/hiv_aids

The economic aspects and implications of AIDS are focused on at www.iaen.org, hosted by the World Bank. To join in email discussions send an email to aids-econ@forumone.com

The Global Reproductive Health Forum South Asia Site seeks to bring together discourses on reproductive health and women's rights that are of particular interest and concern in the South Asian region. www.hsph.harvard.edu/grhf/SAsia

AVERT's website provides information about how to prevent infection with HIV, information for HIV-positive people and the latest news and statistics. Details of AVERT's publications are also included. www.avert.org

The International Council of AIDS Service Organizations (ICASO) is at www.icaso.org

Ahmedabad

Chetna, Lilawatiben Lalbhai's Bunglow, Civil Camp Road, Shahi Bagh, Ahmedabad, Gujarat 380 004. Email chetna@icenet.net and chetna@adinet.ernet.in Contact: Ms Indu Kapoor

Sanchetna, O-45,46, 4th Floor New York Trade Center Thaltej Cross Road Sarkhej, Gandhi Nagar Highway, Ahmedabad, Gujarat 380 054. Contact: Dr Hanif Lakdawala.

Bangalore

Sahodaran, c/o Samraksha, 201 11th Floor, Royal Corner, 182 Lalbagh Road.

Calcutta

Bhoruka Public Welfare Trust, 63 Rafi Ahmed Kidwai Road, Calcutta 700 016. Ph 2448092 or 2449619. Fax 2261196. Email bpwt@cal.vsnl.net.in Contact: Dr Asha Rao.

The Calcutta Samaritans, 48, Ripon Street, Calcutta 700 016. Ph 229 5920 / 9731. Fax 226 8097. Contact: Vijayan Pavamani.

Child in Need Institute or CINI Asha, 63 Rafi Ahmed Kidwai Road, Calcutta 700 016. Ph 4678192, 4671206, 4748063. Fax 2452706. Email ciniasha@giascl01.vsnl.net.in Contact: Ms Sulagna Roy.

Praajak New Alipore Development Society, 468A K Block, New Alipore, Calcutta. Ph 400 0455. Fax 400 0592.

STD/HIV Intervention Programme, 8/2 Bhawani Dutta Lane, Calcutta 700 073. Ph 241-6200. Fax 241 6283.

Vivekananda Education Society, Arcadia, 25/1A Diamond Harbour Road, Calcutta 700 034. Ph 33 468 1550.

Chennai

Ambu Illam or House of Love, Ph 44-4850220. (Counselling and support to men who have sex with men.) Contact: Mr S.Sekhar.

INP+, 29/2, Velu Street, West Mambalam, Chennai 600 033. Ph 44-4744472. Fax 44-4893454. Email inpplus@vsnl.com. Positive Voice newsletter. (*A national network of, for and by people living with HIV/AIDS in India.*) Contact: Mr Ashok Pillai.

Society for AIDS Awareness and Prevention, 31 Hayroon Mansion, 51 Thayar Sahib Street, Anna Salai, Chennai 600 002. Ph 44-4416141 or 4417224. Fax 44-855 1818.

YRG Care, 1 Raman Street, T Nagar, Chennai 600 017. Ph 044-8264242, Fax: 8256842 or 8256900. Email yrgcare@vsnl.com Contact: Ms Suniti Soloman

Delhi

AIDS Bhedbhav Virodhi Andolan (AIDS Anti-Discrimination Movement), P.O. Box 5308, New Delhi 110053.

Michael's Care Home, A-48, Freedom Fighter's Colony, Neb Sarai, New Delhi-110 068. Ph 656 9503

Naz Foundation India Trust, D-45 Gulmohar Park, New Delhi 110 049. Ph 685 1970/1971. Fax 685 9113. Email info@naz.unv.ernet.in

Positive Life, D-2/466 Vasant Kunj. Ph 6893751.

Safdarjung Hospital Model HIV Counselling Centre, Room 542, Fifth Floor, New OPD Block, Safdarjung Hospital. Ph 6198438.

Sahara House, E-453, Greater Kailash-II, New Delhi 110 048. Ph 621 9147. Email sahara@nde.vsnl.net.in

Imphal

Life Line Foundation, P.O.Box No 118, Keishamthong Top Leirak, Imphal 795 001, Manipur. Ph 03852-224186. Contact: Mr N. Vikram Singh.

Social Awareness Service Organisation, RIMS Road (South), Imphal 795 001. Ph 0385-310011. Fax 0385-312230. Email sasoimph@dte.vsnl.net.in. Contact: Mr H. Umesh Sharma.

Kochi

Shramaa, Kolangat House, Pullepady Road, Cochin. Ph 484-354549.

Lucknow

Bharosa Project, 21/6/5 Peerpur House, 8 Tilak Marg, Lucknow. Ph 522-208 689. Email alpana@1w1.vsnl.net.in

Mumbai

AIDS Research & Control Centre (ARCON), Skin and STD Building, Sir JJ Hospital, Mumbai 400 008, India. Ph 22-3742994 or 3742193.

Counselling and Allied Services for AIDS (CASA). Clinic Skin OPD G.T.Hospital, Grandford Market, Mumbai. Ph 4456302, 4445647 or 4361642. Contact: Dr Chitra Subramaniam.

HIV/AIDS Information and Guidance Centre. Suraj Clinic Building 6, Dhruvtara, 90 Feet Street, Ghatkopar East. Ph 5163590 or 5165893.

Humsafar Trust. P.O. Box 6913, Santa Cruz (West), Mumbai 400 054. Voicemail helpline at 9726913. www.humsafar.org. Publish Bombay Dost newsletter. (*Male and gay sexual helpline and drop-in centre for counselling and referral.*)

Indian Health Organisation. RMO's Bungalow, JJ Group of Hospitals, Mumbai 400 008. Ph 3061616 or 3738999.

Lawyers Collective HIV/AIDS Unit, 7/10 Botawalla Building, 2nd Floor, Horniman Circle, Mumbai 400 001. Ph and fax 22-2676213 or 2676219. Email aidslaw@vsnl.com or lawyers@bom2.vsnl.net.in. www.hri.ca/partners/lc. (*Offers legal advice and support to persons living with HIV/AIDS, as well as conducts workshops for lawyers, judges, paralegals, activists, NGOs, GOs, CBOs and of course people with HIV or AIDS.)*

PSI, 149/151 Curson Das Natha Trust Building, Prarthna Samaj, Raja Ram Mohan Roy Road, Behind Khadi Store, Mumbai 400 004. Ph 022-3870883/3894375. Fax 3871415. Email psimumaids@psiindia.com Contact: Ms Shilpa Merchant.

The Salvation Army HIV/AIDS Anonymous Testing and Counselling Centre, 84 Sankhlee Street, Madanpura. Ph 3093556.

Pune

National AIDS Research Institute, Plot No. 73, G Block, MIDC, Bhosari, Pune 411 026. Ph 0212-7121072/7125853/791280/791342/343. Fax 0212-791071 Email hivnet@giaspn01.vsnl.net.in Contact: Mr R.R.Gangakhedkar.

Sangli

Sangram, Kaustabh Bunglow, Chintamani Nagar, Sangli 416 416, Maharashtra. Ph 0233-311644. Contact: Ms Meena Sheshu.

Business leaders interested in taking up HIV/AIDS efforts should contact the Confederation of Indian Industry, Federation of Indian Chambers of Commerce India, ASSOCHAM or the Bengal Chamber of Commerce and Industry, all of which have started programmes in collaboration with NACO.